SCREENING IN HEALTH CARE

Benefit or bane?

SCREENING IN HEALTH CARE

Benefit or bane?

WALTER W. HOLLAND
MD FRCP (Edin) FRCP FRCGP PFPHM

*Department of Public Health Medicine
UMDS, St Thomas's Campus, London*

AND

SUSIE STEWART
MA

*Scottish Forum for
Public Health Medicine, Glasgow*

THE NUFFIELD
PROVINCIAL HOSPITALS
TRUST
1990

Published by the
Nuffield Provincial Hospitals Trust
3 Prince Albert Road, London NW1 7SP
ISBN 0 90057476 3
© Nuffield Provincial Hospitals Trust 1990

Designed by Bernard Crossland
PRINTED IN GREAT BRITAIN BY
BURGESS & SON (ABINGDON) LTD
THAMES VIEW, ABINGDON
OXFORDSHIRE

CONTENTS

ACKNOWLEDGEMENTS

We owe an enormous debt to the following friends and colleagues who have given us their comments on various drafts of the manuscript: Tom Arie, Michael Ashley-Miller, John Colley, Lindsay Davidson, Michael D'Souza, George Forwell, Kathy Helzlsouer, John Horder, Bob Hunter, David Morrell, Roberto Rona, David Stone, Jean Weddell, Bill Williams, Max Wilson, and Charles Wolfe. We are most grateful also to all those we visited and talked to in the United Kingdom, the United States, The Netherlands, and Denmark about specific aspects of screening while preparing the book. The opinions we express are of course entirely our own responsibility. We would also like to thank the President and Library staff of the Royal College of physicians and Surgeons, Glasgow for allowing us to use their excellent library; Beverley Fitzsimons, Susan Giles, Heather Lodge, Maeve O'Connell, and Juliana Oladuti of the Department of Community Medicine at St Thomas' Hospital for editorial, secretarial, and administrative help; and last but not least our families for their encouragement and forbearance.

WALTER HOLLAND
SUSIE STEWART

April 1990

1 SCREENING: A GENERAL VIEW

> Some knowledge of the principles of
> screening and of what it entails in practice
> should form part of the intellectual
> equipment of all concerned with the control
> of disease and the maintenance of health.
> (WILSON AND JUNGNER, 1968)

INTRODUCTION

THAT MEDICINE AND HEALTH CARE HAVE PROGRESSED
dramatically since the beginning of this century can be
seen by glancing at the subjects of papers in the *British
Medical Journal* over the years. In 1900 the concerns
were with topics such as Convalescent Homes for
Soldiers, The Mechanical Origin of Carcinoma, Deaths
from Diarrhoea, Rifle shooting as a National Past-time,
the Insane and their Treatment. In 1940, the *BMJ*
contained papers on topics such as Drug Traffic in
Egypt, Chemotherapy of Gonorrhoea in Women and
Children, Anthracite Dust and Tuberculosis, and Porta-
ble Apparatus for Electrical Convulsions. But even in
1968, the year of publication of the Nuffield Provincial
Hospital Trust's collection of essays entitled *Screening
in Medical Care: Reviewing the Evidence*, volume one of
the *BMJ* contained only three references to screening
—one in relation to anaemia in non-pregnant women,
one on glaucoma, and one on phenylketonuria.

Since then screening has become an extremely popu-
lar concept. Advances in medical skills and technology,
together with increasing knowledge about and expectations of health care among the public bring us into a
very different health arena in 1990 from that in 1968 let
alone 1900. The concept of screening in health care—
that is, actively seeking to identify a disease or pre-
disease condition in people who are presumed and

1

presume themselves to be healthy—is one that now has wide acceptance in our society. In this chapter we would like to take a general view of screening, what we mean by it, what principles we should apply to it, and what criteria should be used for evaluation.

McKeown (1968) defined screening as medical investigation which does not arise from a patient's request for advice for a specific complaint. Screening so defined may have one or more of three main aims and the requirements for its acceptance may be quite different in each case. First it may be the subject of research, for example in the validation of a procedure before it is introduced more widely; secondly, it can be used for the protection of public health—sometimes compulsorily—to identify a source of infection as, for example, with the search for the source of an outbreak of food poisoning; and thirdly, screening can have as its main aim a direct contribution to the health of individuals. It is with the third aim of 'prescriptive' screening that we will deal mainly, although not exclusively, in this book.

SCREENING FOR PREVENTION

Screening stands apart from traditional medicine in that it seeks to detect disease before symptoms present and before an individual decides to seek medical advice. Screening therefore carries considerable ethical responsibilities since it contains the potential to move an individual from the state of supposing himself or herself to be healthy to the state of having some disorder or potential disorder. As Rene Dubos (1960) has pointed out, complete freedom from disease is almost incompatible with the process of living. But we must be sure that screening is not being used to identify conditions that are either untreatable or insignificant since at either end of this spectrum lie anguish and anxiety. As Wald and Cuckle (1989) state:

> Screening must be principally concerned with the prevention of disease and the recognition that it is only

worthwhile screening for disorders which lend themselves to effective intervention.

Simple and obvious as this may sound, it is by no means
always the case although it is, in our view, fundamental
to the integrity of the screening process.

To screen or not to screen?

Opinions in the health professions on the value of
screening remain mixed. Enthusiasts point to the potential for reducing morbidity and mortality. There has
been a resurgence of private screening clinics which
advertise general health screening programmes for men
and women. The new contract for general practitioners
in Britain (Health Departments of Great Britain 1989)
takes its cue from this consumer-led phenomenon and
includes a 'lifestyle check' for newly registered patients, despite the lack of evidence for the efficacy of
this. Particular pressure groups and lay groups, together with the media, may excite a public demand for
screening for a specific condition, often on the basis
of personal experience unsupported by scientific evidence. One fundamental point, raised in the preface to
the previous Nuffield Trust book on screening (1968)
and which remains very relevant today, is the possibility of well-intentioned doctors, patients, and pressure
groups leading a kind of crusade against a particular
disease or diseases and persuading governments to
provide a screening service before a comprehensive
and scientifically respectable assessment of its benefit is
available. In these circumstances the act of screening
runs the risk of acquiring respectability almost by
virtue of its existence. There is, it seems, a tendency to
assume that if you are screened, all will be well. That is
a damaging and dangerous fallacy and every screening
proposal must be rigorously examined against clear
criteria. In the United States, where law suits have been
filed against physicians who failed to detect cancer on
screening, there has been a marked increase in defen-
sive medicine.

Opponents of screening cite that harm it can do in terms of misuse of limited resources, over or misdiagnosis, overtreatment, and the provocation of anxiety and fear. Skrabanek (1988), for example, has re-stated recently his view that 'screening healthy people without informing them about the magnitude of inherent risks of screening is ethically unjustifiable.' Results of one recent study have shown a significant increase in psychological distress in healthy adults who have been screened for coronary heart disease risk factors (Stoate 1989). This author emphasises that advocates of screening tend to assume that the process has only two possible outcomes—benefit or no effect. The possibility that it may actually cause harm is largely ignored. Stoate further argues that

> the debate about who to screen and for what conditions should be widened to take more account of its effect on a person's mental state and subsequent behaviour.

The balance of opinion today seems to lie somewhere between the extremes of enthusiasm and doubt in a cautious and rigorous approach to screening practices and proposals.

Chamberlain (1984) has summarised the benefits and disadvantages of screening and these are shown in Table 1. The benefits are clear. Some patients identified will have an improved prognosis because of early intervention. Disease identified at an early stage may respond to less radical treatment. There should be savings in health service resources by treating diseases before they progress. Those with negative test results can be reassured.

The disadvantages of screening are more complex. They include longer periods of morbidity for patients whose prognosis is unaltered in spite of diagnosis, and overtreatment of insignificant conditions or abnormalities that are identified. In a randomised study of steelworkers with diastolic pressure greater than 95 mmHg, Haynes and colleagues (1978) found that absenteeism from work increased after they had been told

TABLE 1. *Benefits and disadvantages of screening**

BENEFITS	DISADVANTAGES
Improved prognosis for some cases detected by screening	Longer morbidity for cases whose prognosis is unaltered
Less radical treatment which cures some early cases	Overtreatment of questionable abnormalities
Resource savings	Resource costs
Reassurance for those with negative test results	False reassurance for those with false-negative results
	Anxiety and sometimes morbidity for those with false-positive results
	Hazard of screening test

*From Chamberlain (1984) and reproduced by kind permission of the author and publisher.

they had hypertension. 'The increase in illness absenteeism bears a striking relationship to the employee's awareness of the diagnosis but appears unaffected by the institution of antihypertensive therapy or the degree of success in reducing blood pressure.' There are resource costs in finding more illness—in terms of the screening tests themselves, the manpower resources, and the subsequent management of whatever is found. There is the certainty that some individuals with false-negative results will be given unfounded reassurance. Conversely, those with false-positive results will be subjected at the least to needless anxiety and at the worst to unnecessary and disfiguring surgery. Finally there is the question of possible hazard from the screening test itself.

Thus screening should be a hard-headed professional exercise rather than a form of evangelism. Stringent examination of the practice of screening and its implications is essential in any society which takes the health of its citizens seriously. 'The mere existence of unrecognised cases of illness is, by itself, insufficient reason to screen. Disease has many faces, and the hunt is not benign' (Berwick 1985).

Cost, resources, and audit

It is an inescapable fact that, under the present or any foreseeable system, we cannot do everything we might wish in terms of health care. Screening is costly in terms of man hours required to run the programmes, carry out the tests, and act on the results. Limited numbers of skilled professionals are available and this is a problem that will increase in severity as the current demographic changes lead to a smaller work-force. With the explosion of expertise and technology, things are now possible in medicine and health care that were in the realms of science fiction 20 years ago. We have an increasingly informed (and sometimes misinformed!) public who, when made aware of what can be done, expect that it should be available for them and their families. As in other areas of life, we are moving away from the simple quantity issues—routine health care available to all—to the far more complex quality ones—the best and most advanced health care available to all. There is an important change in emphasis from need-led to demand-led health care which has very wide implications. People are also developing a mistrust of high-technology medicine and are demanding more attention to their complex emotional needs.

It is vital, therefore, that there is a proper assessment of the resource implications of any screening or prevention proposal both in terms of primary and of secondary workload, and that screening is included in medical audit. This implies the examination of whether effective, recognised screening has been undertaken as well as consideration of unnecessary ineffective screening procedures. In the South-East London Screening Study (1977), for example, it was found that multiphasic screening increased the work of general practitioners by 10 per cent without a corresponding benefit in health terms. Where a screening test is recommended and available, as for example with screening for cancer of the cervix or breast, this should be considered during the normal medical audit procedure.

Self-responsibility

A properly informed public is a vital and often forgotten ingredient in any analysis of screening. The recent Government White Paper *Working for Patients* recognises this as one of its central themes (Secretaries of State 1989). One of the major weapons in preventive medicine today has to be the persuasion of individuals to take more responsibility for their own health, to seek and accept information on health-damaging and health-enhancing forms of behaviour, and to cooperate in appropriate screening programmes. It is necessary also to keep a sense of balance in the idea of self-responsibility for health. Certainly individuals should be prepared to take reasonable responsibility for their own health. But, given the strong economic, social, political, and environmental influences largely outside the control of the individuals they affect, governments cannot avoid a large measure of collective responsibility for the health of their citizens. It is important too to seek a balance on health awareness. Morbid pre-occupation with health can cause as many difficulties as a lack of awareness of health-damaging behaviours, although, as Acheson (1963) has pointed out, there is little evidence to support the view that the examination of apparently healthy people will turn us into a nation of hypochondriacs. One of the problems with screening is that it does tend to focus on disease rather than health, and it also creates a 'safety-net' philosophy of reliance on the ability of the health professions to identify and solve health problems.

At last in Britain we do seem to be moving towards a more positive concept of health rather than illness, but there is a long way to go. The United States Government has recently set out a list of 21 National Health Objectives for the year 2000 and these are shown in Table 2. They certainly reflect the more aggressive American approach to health care and prevention. At first glance they may also seem too general to be of value, and of course screening is only relevant to those conditions that can be treated. But we in Britain must

TABLE 2. *US Public Health Service national health objectives for the year 2000*

1	Reduce tobacco use
2	Reduce alcohol and other drug abuse
3	Improve nutrition
4	Increase physical activity and fitness
5	Improve mental health and prevent mental illness
6	Reduce environmental health hazards
7	Improve occupational safety and health
8	Prevent and control unintentional injuries
9	Reduce violent and abusive behaviour
10	Prevent and control HIV infection and AIDS
11	Prevent and control sexually transmitted diseases
12	Immunise against and control infectious diseases
13	Improve maternal and infant health
14	Improve oral health
15	Reduce adolescent pregnancy and improve reproductive health
16	Prevent, detect, and control high blood cholesterol and high blood pressure
17	Prevent, detect, and control cancer
18	Prevent, detect, and control other chronic diseases and disorders
19	Maintain the health and quality of life of older people
20	Improve health education and access to preventive health services
21	Improve surveillance and data systems

consider such an approach in order to work towards some cohesion in health care and create a concept of national health priorities, as advocated more than 10 years ago by Stone (1977). There have been recent moves towards this so far as health education and public health are concerned. In England, the Health Education Authority (1989) has recently published a Strategic Plan for the next five years with the objective of ensuring that by the year 2000 people 'are more knowledgeable, better motivated, and more able to acquire and maintain good health'. The Authority designates seven main programmes for health education during the five-year period of the plan (1990–95): HIV/Aids and Sexual Health; Look After Your Heart; Cancer Education; Smoking Education; Alcohol Education; Nutrition Education; Family and Child Health (including immunisation). And the report from an independent multi-disciplinary committee entitled *The Nation's Health: a Strategy for the 1990s* states the belief that a public health strategy should be directed towards three overall health goals—longevity, a good quality of life, and equal opportunities for health (Smith and Jacobson 1988). Members of the committee identified 17 priority areas of action as shown in Table 3. While they claim there is sufficient evidence to merit action in each of these areas, they concede that the evidence is stronger in some cases than others. On the basis of six criteria, they selected 11 of the 17 priorities for which they believe plans for action can currently be justified. These can be grouped into the two main categories of lifestyles for health and preventive services for health, as shown in Table 4. We do regard the setting and stating of national priorities for health as extremely important and will return to this in the final chapter.

TABLE 3. *Priority areas of action in public health strategy**

NUMBER	PRIORITY
1	Reduction of tobacco consumption
2	Promotion of a healthy diet
3	Reduction of alcohol consumption
4	Promotion of physical activity
5	Promotion of road safety
6	Promotion of health at work
7	Effective maternity services
8	Child health surveillance
9	Early cancer detection
10	High blood pressure detection and prevention
11	Reduction of psychoactive drug misuse
12	Services for the elderly
13	Maintenance of social support
14	Promotion of dental health
15	Promotion of a healthy sexuality
16	Adequate income
17	Safe housing

*From *Strategic Plan 1990–95* and reproduced by kind permission of the Health Education Authority.

TABLE 4. *Eleven currently justified priority areas of action in two categories**

LIFESTYLES FOR HEALTH	PREVENTIVE SERVICES FOR HEALTH
Tobacco	Maternity
Diet	Dental health
Physical activity	Immunisation
Alcohol	Early cancer detection
Sexuality	High blood pressure
Road safety	detection

*From *The Nation's Health: A Strategy for the 1990s*. Reproduced by kind permission of the Editors and the King Edward's Hospital Fund for London.

SCREENING AND HEALTH PROMOTION

Screening today is increasingly and inextricably linked with health promotion. One of the major advances in today's concept of screening has been to recognise that it must be concerned not only with identification of disease in its early stages but also with identification of certain types of behaviour which may lead to the development of disease—for example, cigarette smoking, misuse of alcohol, unbalanced or inadequate diet. Some will argue that this is exclusively health promotion and is not the province of screening. But in the context of modern health care it is essential to escape from the compartments of the past and consider health as a whole and the person as an entity rather than as a series of interconnected organs any of which can be diseased in isolation. Thus we will also look at various health promoting activities which have not been traditionally regarded as screening but which fall within the view of screening in prevention as mentioned earlier. One of the strengths of the 1990 contract of service for general practitioners is its emphasis on illness prevention and health promotion as part of routine medical service (Health Departments of Great Britain 1989). Many questions need to be addressed to ensure that screening is used, not as a political football, but as a useful, reliable instrument to improve health care and reduce morbidity and mortality.

In this monograph, we will try to examine the present status of screening in health care in the United Kingdom with research examples as appropriate from elsewhere. We will go on to suggest some ideas for the development of screening in the future, drawing on experience in the United States where the concept of positive health is much more firmly established and where the US Preventive Services Task Force has recently published its *Guide to Clinical Preventive Services* with an assessment of the effectiveness of 169 interventions. We will begin by restating the definitions and principles of screening and its evaluation.

DEFINITIONS

The United States Commission on Chronic Illness Conference on Preventive Aspects of Chronic Disease defined screening as 'the presumptive identification of unrecognised disease or defect by the application of tests, examinations, or other procedures which can be applied rapidly. Screening tests sort out apparently well persons who apparently have a disease from those who probably do not. A screening test is not intended to be diagnostic. Persons with positive or suspicious findings must be referred to their physicians for diagnosis and necessary treatment' (Commission on Chronic Illness 1957).

Various types of screening were defined by Wilson and Jungner (1968). Mass screening is the large-scale screening of whole population groups. Selective screening describes screening of certain selected high-risk groups in the population. Multi-phasic screening encompasses the administration of two or more screening tests to large groups of people (Wilson 1963). Surveillance implies long-term observation of individuals or populations. Case-finding is usually taken to mean screening of patients already in contact with the health service for the main purpose of detecting disease and bringing patients to treatment. The term 'early disease detection' is used to refer to all types of screening in a general sense.

It is important to emphasise the difference between screening where groups of people are invited to attend to be tested and 'opportunistic' screening (Sackett and Holland 1975) where the patient has initiated the health contact and the opportunity is taken to suggest various other appropriate tests, such as the measurement of blood pressure. Since these discussions, it has become apparent that asking simple questions about health behaviour identifies individuals who are at risk and can therefore be legitimately considered under the definition of screening. A good example of this is in chronic bronchitis where the only valid screening test is the question 'do you smoke?' (Colley 1974; Holland 1974).

PRINCIPLES

Despite all the changes in our approaches to health care over the last two decades, the basic principles of screening or early disease detection remain and we make no apology for repeating them here. In reviewing the vast accumulation of publications on screening in recent years, it is obvious that the term is still being used to describe very different processes and without reference to certain fundamental principles.

Wilson and Jungner (1968) summarised these principles as follows:

1. The condition sought should be an important health problem.

2. There should be an accepted treatment for patients with recognised disease.

3. Facilities for diagnosis and treatment should be available.

4. There should be a recognisable latent or early symptomatic stage.

5. There should be a suitable test or examination.

6. The test should be acceptable to the population.

7. The natural history of the disease, including latent to declared disease, should be adequately understood.

8. There should be an agreed policy on whom to treat as patients.

9. The cost of case-finding (including diagnosis and treatment of patients diagnosed) should be economically balanced in relation to possible expenditure on medical care as a whole.

10. Case-finding should be a continuing process and not a 'once for all' project.

Cuckle and Wald (1984) have summarised the basic requirements of a screening programme under eight aspects and these are shown in Table 5.

TABLE 5. *Requirements for a worthwhile screening programme**

ASPECT	REQUIREMENT
1 Disorder	Well-defined
2 Prevalence	Known
3 Natural history	Medically important disorder for which there is an effective remedy available
4 Financial	Cost-effective
5 Facilities	Available or easily installed
6 Ethical	Procedures following a positive result are generally agreed and acceptable both to the screening authorities and to the patients
7 Test	Simple and safe
8 Test performance	Distributions of test values in affected and unaffected individuals known, extent of overlap sufficiently small, and suitable cut-off level defined

*From Cuckle and Wald (1984) and reproduced by kind permission of the authors and publisher.

In the interests of simplicity we have grouped these screening principles into four categories.

Condition. The condition sought should be an important health problem whose natural history, including development from latent to declared disease, is adequately understood. The condition should have recognisable latent or early symptomatic stage.

Diagnosis. There should be a suitable diagnostic test which is available, safe and acceptable to the population concerned. There should be an agreed policy, based on test findings and national standards, as to whom to regard as patients, and the whole process should be a continuing one.

Treatment. There should be an accepted and proven treatment or intervention for patients identified as having the disease or pre-disease condition and facilities for treatment should be available.

Cost. The cost of case-finding (including diagnosis and treatment) should be economically balanced in relation to possible expenditure on medical care as a whole.

EVALUATION

Evaluation of screening is of vital importance and has too often been neglected in the establishment of screening programmes. Screening for cancer of the cervix in the United Kingdom, which we will deal with in more detail in Chapter 6, is one example of a programme that was started without proper provision for adequate scientific evaluation. Once again we make no apology for repeating the list of seven criteria which Cochrane and Holland (1971) suggested for assessment or evaluation of any screening test.

1. Simplicity: a test should be simple to perform, easy to interpret, and, where possible, capable of use by paramedical and other personnel. With increasingly

complex technology certain screening tests, particularly for example in the antenatal and neonatal periods, can only be performed by doctors.

2. Acceptability: since participation in screening is voluntary, a test must be acceptable to those undergoing it.

3. Accuracy: a test must give a true measurement of the condition or symptom under investigation.

4. Cost: the expense of the test must be considered in relation to the benefits of early detection of the disease.

5. Precision or repeatability: the test should give consistent results in repeated trials.

6. Sensitivity: the test should be capable of giving a positive finding when the person being screened has the disease being sought.

7. Specificity: the test should be capable of giving a negative finding when the person being screened does not have the disease being sought.

As Wilson (1963) has stressed, one of the main objections to screening is that tests have frequently been used without knowledge of their scope and limitations. In the early days of screening matters were simpler. The natural history of the conditions being sought, such as tuberculosis and syphilis, was well understood and lines of treatment were clear. The emphasis now is on chronic diseases about which much less is known, and the area of uncertainty is greatest in those conditions which take many years to develop and in which there is no clear boundary between the healthy and the diseased. 'Unless the ground is first cleared by epidemiological studies, it is difficult to see how harm by indiscriminate screening can be avoided' (Wilson 1963).

THE PRESENT MONOGRAPH

Because of the immense scope of the subject, we have divided the present monograph in terms of life-cycle.

We have divided a life-cycle into six screening segments as shown in Table 6. Segment I includes the
antenatal and neonatal periods and infancy. Segment II
deals with childhood. Adolescence and early adulthood, segment III, covers the years 12 to 24. Segments
IV and V contain adult men and women respectively,
and segment V relates to old age.

TABLE 6. *Life-cycle screening segments*

SEGMENT	STAGE OF LIFE	AGE RANGE (yr)
I	Antenatal, neonatal, infancy	−1
II	Childhood	1–11
III	Adolescence and early adulthood	12–24
IV	Adulthood (men)	25–64
V	Adulthood (women)	25–64
VI	Old age	65+

Of course no such classification can be altogether
satisfactory and there will be gaps, overlaps, and
anomalies. The principles for screening and the criteria
for its valuation are, as we have described, well-
established and clear. Our working definition of screening is that it entails inviting an individual for an
examination which may identify a condition at a stage
when it can be treated effectively to inhibit or retard its
development. At some stages of life, however, our
definition of screening has been stretched a little to
cover what purists might consider to be routine clinical
practice. Thus in Chapter 2 we include mention of
measurement of blood pressure or examination of
fundal height of the uterus during pregnancy which
some will claim is simply good medical practice rather
than screening. In Chapter 3, the problem arises as to
what is screening and what is surveillance with the
danger of trying to assess surveillance activities by
screening criteria. Given the broad objectives of health
care in this age group—the identification and if possible

correction of any physical, mental, developmental difficulties and the establishment of good health habits for the future—we would claim that both screening and surveillance are relevant and necessary and too great an insistence on the distinction between them is unrealistic in practice. In Chapters 5 and 6 we have had to make arbitrary decisions on where to include certain conditions such as diabetes, psychiatric disease, and indeed coronary heart disease which affect both men and women.

Because we believe that screening today must attempt to consider the whole person, with the emphasis on health rather than disease, the life-cycle approach, despite its imperfections, is the most practical and realistic. We will consider the present status of screening in each life-cycle segment in certain major diseases or conditions. A number of conditions, such as neuroblastoma and ovarian cancer, have been excluded either because the problem is small in population terms or because there is as yet insufficient evidence of benefit. Other conditions, most notably tuberculosis, are omitted because screening has achieved its objective.

The book is not intended as a comprehensive review of screening for the specialist in any particular field of medicine or health care. Nor is it intended to be a British version of the *US Preventive Services Task Force Report* (1989) which was the product of over four years of intensive efforts by a panel of 20 medical and health experts. Our aim has been to try to pull together the academic and practical strands of screening to provide information for average practitioners, both general and specialist, who can use the text and references to examine in greater detail the basis of our conclusions and draw their own. The book is intended also for health service managers and members of Health Authorities and Boards to try to provide an overview of the current position in screening and highlight some of the present deficiencies and potential strengths of the system.

In considering the state of screening for prevention and health care in the United Kingdom in 1990 two factors seem to stand out. The first is that the has been a clear move away from the concept of general or multiphasic screening which was fashionable 20 years ago. The emphasis now is increasingly on opportunistic screening, screening of high-risk groups, and—with the new contract for general practice—screening for prevention, and this is surely a more sensible approach both in human and financial terms.

The second factor is that there remains wide variation in the provision and standard of screening services throughout the country with too little in the way of quality control or scientific evaluation. There are of course honourable exceptions to these criticisms and some very effective screening is being carried out, as will be shown in subsequent chapters. It is, however, imperative in the next few years that clear national guidelines and standards for any programme of screening are established and monitored and that any screening procedures being continued or started are scientifically evaluated. The designation of one senior person with responsibility for screening in each Health Authority area would be a major step forward in improving co-ordination and efficiency.

In 1971 Cochrane and Holland wrote:

> We believe that there is an ethical difference between everyday medical practice and screening. If a patient asks a medical practitioner for help, the doctor does the best he can. He is not responsible for defects in medical knowledge. If, however, the practitioner initiates screening procedures he is in a very different situation. He should, in our view, have conclusive evidence that screening can alter the natural history of the disease in a significant proportion of those screened.

Thirty years on we would contend that screening by itself can provide no answer to anything. Only if it is carried out efficiently and humanely, leads to an improved outcome in those concerned, and is properly monitored and evaluated should it be contemplated.

REFERENCES

ACHESON, R. M. 'Thoughts on a service for the pre-symptomatic diagnosis of disease'. *Public Health* (1963) 77:261–73.

BERWICK, DONALD, M. 'Scoliosis screening: a pause in the chase'. *Am J Publ Hlth* (1985) 75:1373–4.

CHAMBERLAIN, JOCELYN, M. 'Which prescriptive screening programmes are worthwhile?' *J Epidemiol Comm Hlth* (1984) 38:270–7.

COCHRANE, A. L. AND HOLLAND, W. W. 'Validation of screening procedures'. *Br Med Bull* (1971) 27(1):3–8.

COLLEY, J. R. T. 'Screening for Disease. Diseases of the lung.' *Lancet* 1974, ii:1125–1127.

COMMISSION ON CHRONIC ILLNESS. *Chronic illness in the United States.* Volume 1. Prevention of Chronic Illness. p. 45. Cambridge, Mass: Harvard University Press, 1957.

CUCKLE, H. S. AND WALD, N. J. 'Principles of screening'. In *Antenatal and Neonatal Screening.* N. J. WALD (ed.) Oxford: Oxford University Press, 1984.

DUBOS, RENE, J. *Mirage of Health.* London: George Allen and Unwin, 1960.

HAYNES, R. B., SACKETT, D. L., TAYLOR, D. W., GIBSON, E. S. AND JOHNSON, A. L. 'Increased absenteeism from work after detection and labelling of hypertensive patients'. *New Engl J Med* 1978, 299:741–4.

HEALTH DEPARTMENTS OF GREAT BRITAIN. *General Practice in the National Health Service. The 1990 Contract.* August 1989.

HEALTH EDUCATION AUTHORITY. *Strategic Plan 1990–1995.* London: HEA, 1989.

HOLLAND, W. W. 'Screening for Disease. Taking stock'. *Lancet,* 1974, ii:1494–7.

MCKEOWN, THOMAS. 'Validation of Screening Procedures'. In *Screening in Medical Care: Reviewing the Evidence.* Oxford: Oxford University Press for the Nuffield Provincial Hospitals Trust, 1968.

SACKETT, D. L. AND HOLLAND, W. W. 'Controversy in the detection of disease'. *Lancet,* 1975, 2:357–9.

SECRETARIES OF STATE. *Working for Patients.* White Paper. CM 555. London: HMSO, 1989.

Screening in Medical Care: Reviewing the Evidence. Oxford: Oxford University Press for the Nuffield Provincial Hospitals Trust, 1968.

SKRABANEK, PETR. 'The physician's responsibility to the patient'. *Lancet* 1988, 1:1155–7.

SMITH, A. AND JACOBSON, B. (eds). *The Nation's Health. A Strategy for the 1990's.* A report from an Independent Multidisciplinary Committee chaired by Professor Alwyn Smith. London: King Edward's Hospital Fund for London, 1988.

SOUTH-EAST LONDON SCREENING STUDY GROUP. 'A controlled trial of multiphasic screening in middle age'. *Int. J. Epidemiol.* 1977, 6:357–63.

STOATE, HOWARD, G. 'Can health screening damage your health? *J Roy Coll Gen Practit* 1989,39:193–5.

STONE, DAVID, H. 'Priorities for prevention: a discussion paper'. In *Framework and Design for Planning. Uses of Information in the NHS. Problems and Progress in Medical Care. Essays in Current Research.* London: Oxford University Press for the Nuffield Provincial Hospitals Trust, 1977.

US PREVENTIVE SERVICES TASK FORCE. *Guide to Clinical Preventive Services.* Baltimore: Williams and Wilkins, 1989.

WALD, NICHOLAS AND CUCKLE, HOWARD. 'Reporting the assessment of screening and diagnostic tests.' *Br. Obstet. Gynaecol.* 1989, 96:389–96.

WILSON, J. M. G. 'Multiple screening'. *Lancet* 1963, ii:51–4.

WILSON, J. M. G. AND JUNGNER, G. *Principles and Practice of Screening for Disease.* Geneva: World Health Organization, 1968.

2 ANTENATAL AND NEONATAL SCREENING

> New methods of screening...hold out the
> hope that, with only the rarest exceptions,
> every fetus that is carried to term will be
> born alive with the prospect of surviving
> into adult life physically and biochemically
> whole.
> (SIR RICHARD DOLL, 1984)

INTRODUCTION

THE MONTHS BEFORE BIRTH AND IN THE FIRST YEAR OF
life are those in which most individuals receive more
attention from the health care professions than at any
other time during their lives. As Muir Gray (1984) has
pointed out, most screening services available during
this period are based on sound scientific research and
have been developed rationally. The initial development of a particular technique has normally been
experimental, as a clinical trial, with careful evaluation
and monitoring. These services have therefore been
developed in a much more satisfactory way than many
other current screening procedures which were introduced during the 1950s and 1960s when enthusiasm
was more evident than evaluation (Holland 1974).

ANTENATAL SCREENING

Screening at this stage of life relies increasingly on the
use of complex technology and sophisticated equipment. The advantages of this are that potential problems can be clearly identified. The use of scans rather
than vaginal examinations is less invasive and unpleasant for the woman as well as providing fuller informa-

tion. On the other hand, the spectre of over-testing may be enhanced by the availability of modern equipment which may encourage the routine testing of all pregnant women however healthily and normally the pregnancy is progressing.

Antenatal screening has for many years provided the focus for routine antenatal care which is accepted by most women in the United Kingdom and Western Europe. In order to safeguard the health of the mother and try to ensure the birth of a healthy baby at the most appropriate time, there is an acknowledged programme of care which begins ideally when pregnancy is confirmed. Routine antenatal care in this country at the moment generally consists of a visit to the hospital clinic or general practitioner early in pregnancy, monthly visits up to 30 weeks of pregnancy, fortnightly visits until 36 weeks, then weekly visits until delivery. It is doubtful whether such frequency of visits is necessary in most cases although visits at certain times are clearly desirable. For women who comply, any problems are likely to be detected at an early stage although there remains the question of how to reach those who do not attend and may be most at risk.

Routine antenatal care thus provides a convenient framework and opportunity for screening procedures to be carried out where necessary. There are those who argue that a clear distinction should be made between routine antenatal care and screening for specific fetal abnormalities, and from an academic point of view this is probably so. We would contend, however, that in practical terms this distinction is unrealistic and screening in this period of life can most usefully be seen as a continuum which begins with routine antenatal care and extends as indicated in particular individuals. Antenatal screening tests vary from a simple blood test for anaemia to diagnostic tests for fetal abnormalities, for example, by amniocentesis. They are carried out to check for abnormalities in the pregnancy but only in the last decade has there been any consideration of the woman's perspective. Antenatal screening is a complex and often emotive subject—certain tests may give rise to quite unnecessary anxiety and indeed may actually cause damage. The hazards of amniocentesis, for example, have been investigated (Cuckle and Wald, 1990). Three of four non-randomised studies did not reveal any particular risks (National Institute for Child Health and Development 1976, Medical Research Council of Canada 1977, Crandall *et al* 1980). The fourth study (MRC 1978) suggested a 1·3 per cent excess risk of miscarriage as well as an increased risk of congenital dislocation of the hip, talipes, and neonatal respiratory problems. Results of a more recent large case-control study (Wald *et al* 1983) discount amniocentesis as a cause of congenital dislocation of the hip and talipes although an excess risk of miscarriage of 0·8 per cent was confirmed by the results of a randomised trial (Tabor *et al* 1986, 1988). Since needle size is important in amniocentesis and the trial used a slightly larger size of needle than necessary, Cuckle and Wald (1990) suggest that the excess risk is probably of the order of 0·5 per cent, an estimate confirmed by Mennuti (1989).

As Mennuti (1989) also points out, the relatively advanced gestational age at which amniocentesis is performed and the need to culture amniotic cells before most testing are disadvantages. The delay involved certainly increases the patients' anxiety and if a termination is indicated, there is not only an increased risk to the mother but religious and ethical questions may arise. First trimester chorionic villus sampling is a major step towards earlier, quicker, reliable diagnosis (Rhoads *et al* 1989), although further evaluation is necessary.

Six areas related to the screening process in antenatal care which can pose problems have recently been suggested (Reid 1988). These are availability, knowledge of the test, professional and social support, test procedure, timing of results, the actual results and their aftermath. We will consider each of these briefly here.

Availability

There is considerable variation in the use of antenatal tests—for example, alphafetoprotein (AFP) screening for neural tube defects is more common in Britain than elsewhere in Europe but there are regional variations from one part of the country to another. Certain groups of women, notably those in lower income groups or from ethnic minorities, 'under-use' screening tests (Chamberlain 1984). Thus a test may theoretically be available but not be so in practice. It is also true that some tests have to be carried out before a certain stage in the pregnancy if the results are to be useful. If a woman presents for antenatal care too late, a test which would otherwise have been appropriate may not be available to her—AFP screening, for example, is most accurate between 16 and 20 weeks. Women—particularly those in the lower socio-economic groups who are at particular risk—should, therefore, be encouraged to attend early for antenatal care, should be told about the availability of a particular test, and should be given advice on how it can be helpful to them.

Knowledge of the tests

Many, perhaps most, women experience anxiety during pregnancy as to whether their baby will be normal, and research results have shown that information helps to lessen that anxiety (Macintyre 1981). Many women still appear to lack reasonable information about the antenatal tests they undergo—there remains a tendency for doctors to offer general re-assurance about the test rather than give a full explanation of its purpose. This is particularly so with the more minor routine tests. One of the problems is that available professional time for education and explanation is often inadequate. Women should be told the purpose of a particular test and the actual procedure. The relative risks of the test should also be explained as should the implications of the results. Muir Gray (1984) discusses this problem in relation to screening for neural tube defects. The first test for this is the blood test but what should the pregnant woman be told? She must be given as much information as she wants but constraints are imposed by the amount of time available for discussion. She will obviously be worried by the possibility that her baby may be affected. If the result of the test is positive and the woman decides to undergo amniocentesis and then a termination because of abnormality, the anxiety caused by screening will have been justified. But a high proportion of women have normal test results and their anxiety is unnecessary. Muir Gray further asks how clearly it is explained to women having the blood test that the only effective treatment available if the test is positive is an abortion. It is simple enough to address these issues calmly and objectively in print. But the individual human and ethical complexity of some aspects of antenatal screening requires much more thoughtful study, discussion, and clarification.

Professional and social support

The acceptability of each antenatal screening test depends to some extent on the support available from health professionals and from friends and family. Professional support can be provided in the form of genetic counselling which is important in any discussion of a specific test, risks, and possible results. With amniocentesis however there is not time for referral to a geneticist if an abnormality is detected and responsibility is thus likely to fall on the general practitioner and obstetrician. Some workers have suggested that genetic counselling, however technically proficient, does not always pay sufficient attention to psychological aspects and the emotional aftermath of undergoing such tests (Davies and Doran 1982). This is particularly important in testing for the haemoglobinopathies, which is ideally done before conception, and counselling and support will be needed for some time after the screening test has been carried out.

Test procedure

Even the most routine tests, such as providing samples of blood and urine, are less than pleasant (Macintyre 1981). Again information on the actual procedure and the reason for the test is helpful. Some tests, such as ultrasound where the fetus can be seen, can be a very positive experience. The attitudes and behaviour of those who administer the test are also crucial (Nielson, 1981).

Timing of results

The period between the test and the results has been shown to be a time of great anxiety for women (Nielson 1981, Robinson *et al* 1984). This is particularly so when, as with amniocentesis for example, as long as four to six weeks can elapse between the test and the result. Support is especially important at this time.

Results and their management

The way in which the results are given is very important, whether the news is good or bad (Drillien and Wilkinson 1964). Direct, early, and truthful communication is recommended. Fearn and colleagues (1982) showed that prospective parents told the results of antenatal screening directly by telephone, letter, or in person were less anxious than those left to assume the results by implication. The 'if you do not hear from us within...' method is a sloppy and incomplete means of communication especially on matters of such importance to the individuals concerned.

It is also of course vital that results are properly managed, and the findings of an unpublished study of AFP levels suggest that this is an area where a great deal more scrutiny would be merited (Chapple 1990). In any programme of screening the following questions about results should be capable of being answered without equivocation: How are the results presented —that is, are normal values stated and abnormal results highlighted? Who are the results sent to? Who is responsible for checking on the subsequent care and treatment of those with abnormal results?

There have been suggestions that, in many uncomplicated pregnancies, the number of antenatal visits and tests could be reduced with benefit both to the women concerned and to the workload of those carrying out the examinations and evaluating the samples taken. The antenatal period is also a time of particular importance in screening terms since unnecessary tests and interventions could prejudice the continuation or outcome of the pregnancy. False-positive and false-negative results assume even greater significance in screening at this stage of life when possible termination of pregnancy is at stake. Screening in this context should, therefore, be subject to the most stringent scrutiny.

A European study of antenatal screening found a wide variation in both types of screening procedure routinely practised in different countries and in the number of times some tests were carried out (Heringa and Huisjes 1988). The study covered perinatal and postnatal care also and included a maximum of 10 university hospitals per country. The antenatal screening tests or procedures evaluated in this project, a note on actual practice, and the conclusion of the study on the use of each test are summarised in Table 7. A screening test or procedure was defined as a diagnostic test to be carried out in or offered to all pregnant women accepted for regular antenatal care in one of the participating hospitals, irrespective of risk. There were three possibilities: 1 Not done; 2 Routine; 3 Recommended—that is, either part of normal policy but often omitted in practice or only performed for a special reason.

As can be seen from the comment column, there was a great deal of variation, a number of unnecessary tests, and an urgent need for standardisation, quality control, and re-thinking in this area. One example of this is in screening for gestational diabetes. As the Table shows, 66 per cent of units in the European study did routine screening and 16 per cent recommended doing so.

Universal screening for gestational glucose intolerance during pregnancy is even more strongly advocated in the United States where an oral glucose tolerance test for gestational diabetes mellitus is recommended for all pregnant women between 24 and 28 weeks of gestation (US Preventive Services Task Force 1989). Everett (1989) reports a study which suggests that screening for and treating gestational diabetes may be beneficial but there are not yet sufficient data available to confirm this. However, he questions the importance of universal screening for this condition which only the most affluent societies will be able to afford and suggests that 'since the Second International Workshop Conference on Gestational Diabetes Mellitus has recommended universal screening for gestational diabetes between 24 and 28 weeks of gestation, this has perhaps prematurely come to be the accepted dogma'. The Centers for Disease Control (1986) suggest that if universal screening is not possible, it is advisable to screen women with certain risk factors—age 25 or more, obesity, history of diabetes in a first degree relative, history of pregnancy with stillbirth or infant over 9 lbs, history of congenital malformation in a previous child. The Canadian Task Force (1979) recommends screening pregnant women for gestational diabetes by assessing risk factors and by repeated urine glucose testing. However, in a recent review of the evidence, Ales and Santini (1989) showed that the scientific data supporting universal screening in this context are at best limited. They suggest that, until the evidence can be extended beyond that on infant birthweight, a more restrained approach than universal screening may be appropriate.

In Britain, as Jarrett (1984) has pointed out, establishing whether a woman has pre-existing diabetes and her management if she has, is part of normal clinical practice. Formal antenatal screening is therefore not involved. Identifying women with gestational diabetes would involve screening. But in the absence of clear evidence that gestational diabetes carries an extra risk to the fetus, and in the absence of evidence that, if a risk did exist, an effective treatment was available, there is, in our view, no case for routine screening for this condition.

There are also differing opinions about antenatal screening for asymptomatic bacteriuria (Campbell-Brown *et al* 1987). In the European study, only 54 per cent of respondents performed this routinely (Table 7). However, in view of the simplicity of the test and its potential usefulness in preventing low birthweight, fetal and neonatal mortality, and the onset of acute pyelonephritis in pregnancy we would suggest that it should be part of routine antenatal screening.

TABLE 7. *Antenatal screening tests or procedures evaluated in the European study**

TEST	ACTUAL PRACTICE	CONCLUSIONS
Vaginal examination	Routinely done at first visit. Not normally repeated.	Largely replaced by scan. Validity doubtful and procedure itself may not be harmless
Fundal height	Predictive value of this test for detecting the growth retarded fetus is about 50%. For measurement of fundal height (cm), a sensitivity of 64–86% and a specificity of 75–95% have been reported. About half of respondents measured fundal height in cm, a quarter estimate using landmarks of the body, and one-	Efficacy of screening for intrauterine growth retardation is hard to assess. There is no generally accepted definition and in most cases no effective treatment is available. Intensive monitoring in suspected cases may prevent hypoxia. Measurement in cm is the best method but a single method

TABLE 7.—*continued*

TEST	ACTUAL PRACTICE	CONCLUSIONS
Fundal height—*continued*	third measure uterine size directly in weeks.	with a higher predictive value is required.
Breast examination	Breast examination, as part of antenatal screening to detect abnormalities and disorders that could interfere with the mother's health or with breast feeding, was routinely performed by 51% of clinicians.	Routine breast examination in early pregnancy, with emphasis on information and education about self-examination and breast-feeding, may seem advisable but there is no scientific support for this.
Blood pressure and proteinuria	All responding clinicians checked blood pressure at each visit and 91% screened for proteinuria at almost every visit.	Benefits of these tests are hard to quantify but they should be continued as serious complications can occur in a risk group that can be identified with little effort. Agreement needs to be reached on standardisation of BP measurement and diagnostic criteria to minimise over-diagnosis.
Cervical smear	Routinely performed by 63% of respondents and recommended by a further 33%. In some countries it is compulsory.	There is little information about either the prevalence of cervical disorder in pregnancy or the validity or efficacy of screening. Screening all pregnant women may result in a relatively high

Table 7.—*continued*

TEST	ACTUAL PRACTICE	CONCLUSIONS
Cervical smear— *continued*		false-positive rate in the younger age groups. As invasive diagnostic tests following a positive result may not be harmless in pregnancy, are likely to cause anxiety and consume limited resources, caution is required. Using a lower age limit for screening of 25 years, the workload would be almost halved and the detection rate would still be 92%.
Weight	A very wide range of weight gain is compatible with clinical normality. In this study, 98% of clinicians weighed their patients at each visit.	Weight gain may be helpful in diagnosing other signs or symptoms of pathological conditions and is relatively simple to measure. However, the criteria used to judge the values and the consequences of abnormal findings are unclear.
Blood group typing	All participating units performed ABO blood group typing routinely. In 64 units the Rhesus(D) typing was included.	Since haemorrhage associated with pregnancy and labour is still one of the main causes of maternal death, screening by blood group typing of the mother should be done routinely.

TABLE 7.—*continued*

TEST	ACTUAL PRACTICE	CONCLUSIONS
Haemoglobin, haematocrit, ferritin, haemoglobin-opathies	Over 90% of respondents measured Hb at least once and many more often. Only about 4% measured neither Hb nor haematocrit. Ferritin assessments were performed routinely by only 9% of units. 19% of clinicians routinely screen for haemoglobino-pathies with a blood test. In Italy and Greece, with high prevalence of thalassaemia, all clinics at least recommend screening.	Without iron supplementation anaemia is a common disorder in pregnancy. In addition to acquired anaemia, some regions of S. Europe have a high prevalence of hereditary structural Hb disorder. Thus there is reason for antenatal screening for anaemia although the efficacy of screening has not been evaluated. Three major reasons are usually put forward for antenatal screening for the haemoglobin-opathies (Stein 1984): (i) it can help to avoid inappropriate treatment in case of anaemia. (ii) it can enable identification of high-risk pregnancies for surveillance; and (iii) it can help to identify cases where the partner should be screened and antenatal diagnostic tests suggested.

TABLE 7.—*continued*

TEST	ACTUAL PRACTICE	CONCLUSIONS
Syphilis	Almost all (97%) respondents performed screening routinely on first visit. As a recent infection may be missed or infection may be acquired during pregnancy, some repeat the test in the last trimester.	A syphilitic infection during pregnancy will have such serious consequences, serological screening tests should be compulsory in antenatal care.
Toxoplasmosis	Routine screening was performed by only 34% of clinicians in the study, mainly in Italy, Belgium and France.	Serological screening may help in primary prevention by finding women without antibodies who are at risk from infection. Screening in a low prevalence population not recommended.
Rubella	Most (91%) responding clinicians either recommended a serological test for rubella or performed it routinely.	Antenatal screening aimed at primary and secondary prevention should continue. Termination of pregnancy is generally advised when a first-trimester infection is diagnosed.
Cytomeg-alovirus (CMV)	Only 12% of respondents reported routine screening for CMV and there was no information about methods used or action taken.	Diagnosis is difficult, especially during pregnancy, and the predictive value of serological screening is uncertain. Further, there is no effective treatment. At

TABLE 7.—*continued*

TEST	ACTUAL PRACTICE	CONCLUSIONS
Cytomeg-alovirus (CMV)—*continued*		present there is no evidence to support routine screening for CMV.
Listeria	Only 9% of respondents routinely perform screening and there was no information on the nature of tests or consequences of a positive result.	No laboratory screening test is available to identify those at risk of complications from a listeria infection. Clinical judgment is therefore the best screening procedure to identify suspected cases.
Group B beta-haemolytic streptococci (GBBHS)	Only 13% of clinicians routinely performed antenatal screening and these mainly in special cases.	There are no grounds for routine antenatal screening because the predictive value of the test is very low and there is doubt as to the effectiveness of the intervention.
Asymptomatic bacteriuria	54% of respondents routinely perform antenatal screening for bacteriuria. About 25% do not, and others use history as a first screening.	Further research is required. There is much controversy about this in published reports.
Hepatitis B virus (HBV)	Only 36% of respondents routinely performed a serological screening test on HBV. Some 20% recommended it in suspected high-risk groups.	Highly sensitive laboratory tests are available for serological screening. For the protection of newborn a serological screening test at

TABLE 7.—*continued*

TEST	ACTUAL PRACTICE	CONCLUSIONS
Hepatitis B virus (HBV)— *continued*		least once in the late third trimester would be sufficient. Screening at first antenatal visit would be advisable to prevent transmission of HBV to other individuals (infant and health care workers) during pregnancy and labour. The cost-effectiveness of screening and intervention very much depends on the prevalence of HBV in the population. There is insufficient evidence to suggest routine antenatal screening in low-prevalence populations.
Ultrasound	82% of respondents routinely perform ultrasound, irrespective of obstetric risk	Ultrasound is a valuable diagnostic test in pregnancy when performed on specific indications. However, its usefulness as a routine screening procedure in the general pregnant population has not been sufficiently demonstrated. Its use as a first screening procedure is time-consuming, and

TABLE 7.—*continued*

TEST	ACTUAL PRACTICE	CONCLUSIONS
Ultrasound— *continued*		may produce a high rate of false positives. Fundamental research is a priority.
Cardio-tocography	25% of respondents performed the non-stress test (NST) routinely (a majority of clinicians in Belgium, Italy and Germany). Of the 34% of units which recommended the test in certain circumstances, most did so in post-term pregnancies or during labour.	NST is not a well-standardised test method and its reproducibility and validity are limited. The need for repeat testing will be high and there will also be a risk of unnecessary intervention. The incidence of effects attributable to fetal distress in the general population is very low and the efficacy of screening is not proven even in a high-risk population. Routine screening by NST is not recommended.
Fetal movements	64% of units routinely checked fetal movements—84% of them did this by casual enquiry.	Further research is needed. Evaluation of fetal movements is a relatively simple test to identify the fetus at risk of intrauterine death but it is a difficult and unsystematic area at present. Basic research is in progress to study the qualitative

TABLE 7.—*continued*

TEST	ACTUAL PRACTICE	CONCLUSIONS
Fetal movements— *continued*		aspects of fetal movements by ultrasound.
Placental functions	Only 22% of respondents performed placental function tests (PFTs) on a routine basis; a further 19% recommended doing so in specific circumstances.	The main aim of these tests seems to have been to identify IUGR and development of more direct measurements such as fetal ultrasound is likely to make this redundant. Even at present, routine PFT screening in a population irrespective of risk cannot be recommended.
Coagulation disorders	Nine per cent of respondents performed a screening test on coagulation disorders and 34% recommended it in high-risk pregnancies or when epidural analgesia would be offered during labour.	In general these disorders are so rare that widespread laboratory screening could not be justified. Patient and family history and a physical examination should be the first screening procedures.
Maternal serum AFP (SAFP)	28% of respondents performed SAFP screening for neural tube defects, 25% recommended doing so, and 39% did not.	This is an important screening measurement aimed at identifying pregnancies at sufficient risk of NTD to justify diagnostic tests. The outcome of a screening

TABLE 7.—*continued*

TEST	ACTUAL PRACTICE	CONCLUSIONS
Maternal serum AFP (SAFP)— *continued*		programme can be that over 3/4 of all cases of open spina bifida and nearly all cases of anencephaly can be detected with a very low false-positive rate. In practice, the effectiveness of such programmes have been shown to be less impressive.
Gestational diabetes	66% of units did routine screening and 16% recommended doing so. Of these 65% screened with a test on glucosuria.	In practice there seems to be no settled policy on screening for gestational diabetes. The consequences of the disease for mother and child are hard to quantify. At present no definite advice can be given on whether routine antenatal screening should be done. Recent evidence suggests that more research is needed.

* From Heringa and Huisjes (1988) and reproduced by kind permission of the authors.

Another area of debate is antenatal screening for human immunodeficiency virus (HIV) which we will discuss more fully in Chapter 4. There is no national policy on this in the United Kingdom at the moment. However January 1990 saw the start of a programme of anonymised testing for HIV in England and Wales run by the Medical Research Council. Initially, excess blood taken from patients attending specified antenatal and genitourinary clinics will be tested for the virus and screening will later be extended to general hospital patients and to Guthrie tests in the neonatal period. Patient identifiers will be removed before testing with only gender, age, and location retained. Patients will not be asked individually for consent but will know of their clinic's policy and may opt out. This is seen as an important step in understanding the epidemiology of HIV (Gill, Adler, and Day 1989), although ethical reservations have been expressed (Gillon 1987).

We would now like to consider antenatal screening in three groups of conditions which are well documented and which illustrate many of the problems encountered in screening at this stage of life—Down syndrome, the haemoglobinopathies, represented by thalassaemia major, and neural tube defects.

DOWN SYNDROME

Down syndrome is the most common cause of severe congenital mental retardation in the United Kingdom. The only current routinely available preventive measure is antenatal diagnosis by amniocentesis, followed by termination of affected pregnancies (Stone, Rosenberg, and Womersley 1989). This has its limitations—the sensitivity of the test is low and success is strongly dependent on the availability of adequate diagnostic facilities and a good acceptance rate among eligible women (Goujard 1988). However, the same practice prevails in the United States where other methods are still considered to be at the research stage (US Preventive Services Task Force 1989). The Task Force Report recommended that amniocentesis for karyotyping should be offered to pregnant women aged 35 years or above. They also suggested that maternal serum alphafetoprotein should be measured on all pregnant women during weeks 16–18 where adequate facilities for counselling and follow-up are available. They do not regard ultrasound as a routine screening test for congenital defects at present.

In a study of recent trends in the prevalence and secondary prevention of Down syndrome, Stone and colleagues (1989) found that antenatal diagnosis appears to have made little impact on the birth prevalence of the condition in Glasgow. This they attribute partly to the failure to extend amniocentesis to more than a minority of older pregnant women, and partly to the larger number of Down syndrome babies being born to younger women, supposedly at low risk. On the basis of these results, even if all pregnant women aged 35 years and over underwent amniocentesis, the birth prevalence of Down syndrome would be reduced by only 35 per cent at best. These workers suggest that there is a need for further aetiological research, for continued epidemiological monitoring, for an improvement in the relatively low uptake of amniocentesis by older mothers, and for the development of a screening test which can be offered to the whole of the pregnant population.

The possibility of improving the effectiveness of antenatal screening for Down syndrome by measuring human chorionic gonadotrophin concentrations in maternal serum during the second trimester to select women for diagnostic amniocentesis has been examined by Wald and colleagues (1988). The median maternal serum human chorionic gonadotrophin concentration in 77 pregnancies associated with Down syndrome was twice that in 385 unaffected pregnancies matched for maternal age, gestational age, and duration of storage of serum sample. Measuring human chorionic gonadotrophin in maternal serum was an effective screening test which gave a lower false-positive rate (3 per cent) at a 30 per cent detection rate than that for maternal age (5 per cent) and the two existing serum screening tests, unconjugated oestriol (7 per cent) and alphafetoprotein (11 per cent). The most effective screening results were achieved by combining all four variables—at the same 30 per cent detection rate, the false-positive rate fell to 0.5 per cent. This screening method would detect over 60 per cent of affected pregnancies, more than double that achievable with the same amniocentesis rate in existing programmes, and could reduce the number of affected children born annually in the United Kingdom from about 900 to about 250. Antenatal screening programmes using maternal age in conjunction with the three biochemical markers would also be cost-effective. Alphafetoprotein is already likely to be performed routinely as part of antenatal screening for neural tube defects. The extra cost of the tests for human chorionic gonadotrophin and unconjugated oestriol would be less than the cost of the amniocentesis and karyotyping that would be necessary to obtain the same rate of detection. Wald and colleagues further suggest that it might be possible to improve the effectiveness of maternal serum screening further by ultrasound screening to measure fetal femur length as a complementary technique although studies of the correlation between femur length and the serum markers would have to be done.

In a further examination of screening for Down syndrome, Cuckle and Wald (1990) point out that the use of maternal serum markers is likely to be generally acceptable to both the women and the laboratories concerned. From the point of view of the former, it involves no additional inconvenience since the tests can be carried out on a blood sample already collected routinely; and for laboratories it merely involves the performance of two additional tests already available for other purposes. In addition, computer software for interpretation of the screening data obtained is now available commercially.

Reservations had earlier been expressed about this approach. In 1987 the American College of Obstetricians and Gynecologists took the view that the measurement of alphafetoprotein levels as a screening test for Down syndrome is still at the investigatory stage. Elias and Annas (1987) supported this view and advised caution over the claim that ultrasound can identify fetuses with Down syndrome on the basis of a thickened nuchal skinfold and relatively short femur. From the point of view of the women involved, Marteau and colleagues (1988) stressed the necessity of ensuring

adequate counselling and explanation before the introduction of any new screening tests into routine obstetric
care to minimise the distress now known to arise for the
women involved.

We would agree in general with Cuckle and Wald
(1990) that the additional use of maternal serum
markers is likely to be acceptable to the women
concerned, would not cause unnecessary laboratory
overload, and should be considered.

THALASSAEMIA MAJOR

The genetic disorders of haemoglobin structure and
synthesis are probably the most common single gene
disorders in the world and constitute a major public
health problem in some countries and some ethnic
groups. The US Preventive Services Task Force (1989),
for example, recommended that haemoglobin analysis
should be performed routinely at the first prenatal visit
on all pregnant black women.

The World Health Organisation (WHO) attaches
great importance to thalassaemia which is a very
widespread condition in certain areas and a considerable health problem worldwide. It is common in the
Mediterranean area and in the Middle and Far East. In
Britain it occurs mainly among Cypriots and Asians,
less commonly among Chinese and Italians, and rarely
among the indigenous British (WHO 1982). Thalassaemia can also be used as a model genetic condition to
demonstrate general approaches for the control of
congenital disorders. It heads the list for avoidable
inherited conditions—the technology is available and
prevention is sought by most at-risk communities and is
highly cost-effective. In principle, with a combination of
prospective heterozygote diagnosis and fetal monitoring almost all births of infants with thalassaemia could
be prevented (Kuliev 1988).

Thalassaemia major is a prime candidate for screening before conception. Screening by blood tests for the

presence of the thalassaemia carrier state permits the identification of prospective parents at risk of having children with the condition. As Petridou and Loukopoulos suggest (1988), screening should be incorporated as part of an individual's routine health care with genetic counselling provided for those found to be positive. Other opportunities arise during the antenatal and neonatal period, as well as later in life—for example, during sponsored ethnic community programmes, for recruits to military service, immigrants and refugees at the time of first arrival into the host country.

It does raise various questions from the patient's point of view as Matthews (1988) points out in the following quote from an adult thalassaemia patient.

> Physicians are patients' guardians of health but not of choice or conscience... Patients must be given all available knowledge to aid them in the correct choice of treatment that best suits them. Freedom of choice is paramount to the maintenance of human dignity.

The lowest fall in the birth-rate of infants with thalassaemia major in different control programmes has been in the United Kingdom (Modell and Petrou 1988). There are at least three reasons for this. One is the large size of population; the second is that the haemoglobinopathies occur mainly in ethnic minorities scattered throughout a larger indigenous population that is not at risk; and thirdly, one of the largest of such groups has been the first generation Muslim immigrants from rural areas of Pakistan, most of whom find the concept of midtrimester diagnosis and abortion socially and morally unacceptable. In Britain the group most affected by thalassaemia used to be British Cypriots living in North-East London. In 1980 Modell, Ward and Fairweather reported that almost 100 per cent of at-risk British Cypriot couples counselled had asked for fetal testing. This particular community is now well informed about thalassaemia and its implications for the future of the expected child and most couples expect to be screened. Thus, because of changing immigration trends and differential uptake of fetal testing, British Asians are now the group most affected (Modell *et al* 1984). Muslims from Pakistan now produce about half of the thalassaemic children born annually in the United Kingdom, and only about 20 per cent of couples at risk in this group have currently been able to accept fetal testing. Given certain moral and religious objections to termination of pregnancy in this group, as mentioned above, any extension of screening coverage is likely to be difficult but efforts should be made.

As Modell and colleagues (1984) point out, one of the main reasons for the small effect of fetal testing on the thalassaemia birth-rate in Britain is a lack of prospective heterozygote screening and appropriate genetic counselling. There is no uniform national policy for heterozygote diagnosis. No one group of health professionals has yet taken responsibility for the organisation of screening—although it has been suggested that the appropriate group might be the regional clinical geneticists (Modell *et al* 1984). Finally there does need to be better communication with the ethnic minorities, in particular the Pakistani Muslims, to explain the implications of the condition and alert them to the possibility of antenatal, and ideally pre-conception, testing.

Recently, earlier fetal diagnosis based on chorionic villus sampling and gene mapping (Old *et al* 1982, Weatherall *et al* 1985) has begun to be introduced in the United Kingdom and this may hold the key to future improvements in this area. The critical question is whether the transfer of diagnosis from the second to the first trimester of pregnancy will increase the acceptability of the procedure to those most at risk. Although precise figures are not available, Modell and Petrou (1988) have the impression that first trimester fetal diagnosis is acceptable to about 80 per cent of British Pakistani couples who know about the condition because they already have an affected child. It is impossible at present to predict whether this would be true of prospectively diagnosed couples at risk.

For thalassaemia there is, therefore, an urgent need for a co-ordinated national policy of information, counselling, and antenatal screening aimed at at-risk groups. Ideally, as we have said, this process should take place before conception. It is also imperative to ensure that satisfactory continuing support and surveillance with appropriate prophylactic treatment are available for affected individuals. Milne (1990), in a retrospective study of the care of children with sickle cell disease, found that treatment and follow-up were inadequate and erratic. His findings are important in reinforcing the message that screening will not achieve its full potential without a systematic programme that links follow-up with diagnosis.

NEURAL TUBE DEFECTS

Four main types of neural tube defect can be identified —anencephaly, spina bifida, encephalocele and iniencephaly—anencephaly and spina bifida account for around 90 per cent of all cases (Eurocat 1986). The prevalence of NTD remains much higher in the British Isles than in continental Europe with geographical variations within the country (Elwood and Elwood 1980).

Intervention based on antenatal screening and diagnosis, followed by termination of affected pregnancies, is at present the only proven way of preventing NTD (Goujard 1988). This is based on the detection of raised levels of alphafetoprotein in the maternal serum or amniotic fluid or both, in early pregnancy. In all cases the optimal time for screening is between 16 and 18 weeks of pregnancy (UK Collaborative Study 1977). More recently, antenatal ultrasound examination has been considered as an alternative in some centres.

There are two possible strategies. The first is to screen high-risk cases with a previously affected child or a positive family history. However, in the British

Isles this would detect only 5 per cent of cases in the population since there is no simple maternal variable, such as age, to identify an at-risk group in the general population. The second strategy is total population screening, attempting to cover each pregnancy.

In Britain, in view of the high prevalence of NTD, the cost of screening appears cheap (Wald and Cuckle 1984) and its practice is well developed. AFP maternal serum screening is the primary screening test with ultrasonography in those with raised levels of AFP. The selection of a cut-off level (Wald 1984) must be a compromise based on the resources available to carry out ultrasound examination and amniocentesis. As already mentioned, it is also essential that results are properly managed. To detect small neural tube defects, focused ultrasound may be necessary and this will require the availability of the necessary equipment and highly trained staff. Thus the use of AFP testing requires high quality medical and laboratory work and good availability of follow-up and is probably best concentrated at a small number of specialist centres. Goujard (1988) cautions against uncontrolled extension of antenatal screening for neural tube defects since this would increase the risk of errors.

Better co-ordination and organisation of screening programmes in this area is vital.

> The present challenge in AFP screening is organisa-
> tional. While in many places, ad hoc screening arrange-
> ments have proved to be satisfactory, it has become
> apparent that health authorities have not been uniformly
> successful at initiating, delivering, and monitoring pro-
> grammes effectively (Wald and Cuckle 1984).

Stone and colleagues (1988), in a study of screening for congenital neural tube defects over the period 1974–85 found that screening resulted in the termination of a larger proportion (59 per cent) of anencephalic than spina bifida (23 per cent) pregnancies. This was mainly because of the greater sensitivity of serum-alphafetoprotein screening for the former defect. Any improvement in the efficacy of screening for spina bifida will therefore require either an increase in the sensitivity of the test or an increase in the proportion of the pregnant population screened, or preferably both. It is also worth emphasising the importance of separating the impact of screening on anencephalus and spina bifida since the former is an invariably fatal condition.

The practical implications of these findings are described as threefold (Stone *et al* 1988). Firstly, because the prevalence of both defects might have shown a natural decline as elsewhere in Britain in the absence of screening (OPCS 1983; Carstairs and Cole 1984), aetiological and other research should continue to try to explain the phenomenon. Secondly, continuous public health monitoring of the prevalence of both defects is essential since the population must be considered vulnerable to a future increase in frequency. Thirdly, since the only effective preventive response to the problem of neural tube defects is antenatal screening, this should be continued in areas, such as the West of Scotland, considered to be at high risk.

The question of whether we can afford screening for neural tube defects has also been raised. In a study in South Wales, Hibbard and colleagues (1985) estimated the clinical and financial gains and losses from five different options for screening for open neural tube defects. As well as estimating the overall clinical costs of a screening service, they showed that if the prevalence, including terminations, of open neural tube defects is between 1·25 and 5 per 100 births, the financial cost of avoiding the birth of a seriously handicapped child who would survive for more than 24 hours is in the range £9000 to £54,000, depending on the option adopted and the prevalence of the condition in the target population. Prevalence was the biggest determinant of cost. They suggest that their data could provide a basis for assessment and discussion of resource priorities in the National Health Service. They further state their view that further development of serum-alphafetoprotein screening should be discouraged in areas with a prevalence of neural tube defects below 2·5 per 1000 until some notion of maximum acceptable cost to the National Health Service has been agreed.

SUMMARY

Screening in the antenatal period, in terms of routine antenatal care, is relatively well organised for those who present themselves. There is clearly scope, however, for improving communication and information provided when further tests are indicated, and for improving efforts to reach those who do not present themselves but who may be most in need of attention at this time.

In the specific conditions considered here the position is variable. With Down syndrome the current almost universal screening method remains diagnostic amniocentesis on the basis of maternal age. We would hope that, with further work on the evaluation of screening by amniocentesis in conjunction with the three maternal serum markers described earlier, this may come to be the screening method of choice in the near or foreseeable future. With thalassaemia, screening strategy should certainly concentrate on testing high-risk groups. Efforts now must focus on improving organisation, increasing uptake, particularly for example in British Asians, and providing appropriate information, advice, treatment, and follow-up for those affected. We would agree with Stone and colleagues (1988) that, despite the natural decline in the prevalence of neural tube defects, serum-alphafetoprotein screening should be continued in high-risk areas as the only effective preventive response to the problem. The prevalence point at which populations cease to be considered at high-risk remains open to debate. Screening for this group of defects appears to vary considerably from one area of the country to another, and better co-ordination, organisation, and evaluation are essential.

NEONATAL SCREENING

Screening procedures in the period immediately after birth and in the first 12 months of life, as well as throughout childhood, were reviewed comprehensively by the Hall Committee (1989). They divided tests into six categories—Clinical Examinations, Laboratory and Radiological Tests, Growth Monitoring, Tests of Vision, Hearing, and Development. They then looked at each test or procedure and recommended whether it should be continued or introduced (C), was of uncertain benefit and required further evaluation (U), or should be discontinued or not introduced (D). Their findings are summarised in Table 8 and we will look at them briefly here in relation to the neonatal period.

In the clinical examination category, Hall's Working Group recommended that screening for hypertension should be discontinued. The yield of secondary hypertensives is very low and optimum management of primary hypertension in children has not been clearly defined. Similarly with asthma, the report emphasises that an increasing awareness of the high prevalence of mild asthma is more useful than a formal screening programme.

With undescended testes, they observe that three out of four testes undescended at birth are normally descended by three months. The second examination at 8–9 months is important since treatment before 18 months may improve the prognosis for fertility.

In the section on laboratory and radiological tests, Hall and his group highlighted three groups of tests which await further evaluation. Those for inborn errors of metabolism are still under investigation. With cystic fibrosis better tests may soon be available using DNA technology and these would open the way for antenatal diagnosis in affected families. Measurement of blood cholesterol and lipids in children from families with familial hypercholesterolaemia or a history of early ischaemic disease may be useful but also requires further evaluation.

TABLE 8. *Summary of screening procedures in six categories in the antenatal and neonatal periods with the Hall Report recommendations on status**

CONDITION	SCREENING PROCEDURE	AGE FOR TEST	STATUS**
I			
Clinical			
Examination			
CDH	Ortolani/Barlow manoeuvre	Birth	C
	Classic signs	10 days	
	Ortolani/Barlow manoeuvre	6 weeks	C
	Classic signs	6 weeks	C
	Reduced abduction	6–9 months	C
CHD	Clinical examination	2–10 days	C
	Auscultation	+	
		6–8 weeks	
		(+once between	
		8 weeks and 5 years)	
Hypertension	Blood pressure measurement	Any	D
Asthma	Questionnaire on wheezing	Any	D
Undescended testes	Clinical examination	2–10 days	C
	Clinical examination	8–9 months	C

II Laboratory and Radiological Tests			
PKU	Guthrie	7 days	C
Hypothyroidism	T4/TSH	7 days	C
Inborn errors of metabolism	Biochemical tests	7 days	U
Cystic fibrosis	Stool trypsin etc	Birth	U
Duchenne muscular dystrophy	Creatine phosphokinase	Birth	D
Haemoglobino-pathies	Sickle test Hb analysis	Birth	C
Familial hyper-cholesterolaemia	Blood cholesterol and lipids	Any	U
III Growth Monitoring			
Failure to thrive	Weighing	Birth All clinic visits 0–1 year On request	C

TABLE 8.—*continued*

CONDITION	SCREENING PROCEDURE	AGE FOR TEST	STATUS**
Abnormally large or small head	Measurement of head circumference	2–10 days	C
		6 weeks	C
IV Vision			
Congenital cataract	Red reflex	Birth	C
Other causes of partial sight and blindness	Family history Observation	Birth + 6 weeks	C
Squint	Manifest cover test	8 months	D
V Hearing			
Sensori-neural hearing loss	Neonatal screening	Birth	D
	Distraction test	7–9 months	C
VI Developmental Impairments			
Neurodevelopmental problems and psychiatric disorders			D

* Adapted from *Health for All Children* (Hall 1989) and reproduced by kind permission of the authors and Oxford University Press.
** C=Continue or introduce; U=Uncertain, needs further evaluation; D=Discontinue or do not introduce.

In regard to growth monitoring, the Report recommends the continuation of the current practice in terms of weight, height, and head circumference while noting that this is an under-evaluated area.

In their analysis of screening for defects of vision, members of the group recommend discontinuation of the manifest cover squint at 8 months. They observe that an awareness that squinting is abnormal is important and parents and professionals should inspect eyes frequently. Formal screening by people other than orthoptists is not recommended. With hearing, they caution that the distraction test at 7–9 months is potentially misleading if not properly performed. Parental suspicion must be taken seriously and parents should be asked about hearing at every opportunity.

We regard the Hall Report as an extremely valuable assessment of health care in infancy and childhood. It is perhaps worth stressing here too that some factors which are difficult to measure scientifically and which often rely on the experience and intuition of the good general practitioner or other member of the practice team must not be lost sight of (Morrell 1990). The neonatal period is undoubtedly a time when the general practitioner is in a good position to observe and assess the baby and the family within the general framework of routine health care and without intrusion, and this is very important. Regular measurements of height and weight gain should be charted—a sudden change in weight gain, for example, is a very valuable indication that something may be wrong. Similarly, regular observation of the mother/child relationship and how the new baby has affected the dynamics of the whole family, may be crucial to the infant's development although difficult to measure objectively or scientifically. Simple items such as a baby's ability to sit at 6–7 months and so on can help to indicate those at risk.

We would now like to consider four conditions or groups of conditions relevant in the neonatal period which illustrate the spectrum of value of screening. Screening for phenylketonuria and more recently congenital hypothyroidism can be considered two of screening's success stories, well established and accepted by most as worthwhile. Screening for congenital dislocation of the hip remains the subject of much controversy, not least because it has been suggested that the screening procedure can cause the damage it is intended to detect. Finally, formal screening procedures for developmental disorders in the neonatal period, and indeed throughout childhood, which the Hall Committee suggested should be discontinued.

PHENYLKETONURIA

Testing for phenylketonuria (PKU) is the most accepted form of neonatal screening within the European Community and covers more than 90 per cent of the newborn population in 16 countries (Schmidt 1986). In the United States routine screening for PKU is required in all newborn babies in every state (Stevens, Rigilano, and Wilson 1988; US Preventive Services Task Force 1989). The birth prevalence of the condition is around 11 per 100,000 babies screened although there are variations within and between countries.

This condition is a prime candidate for screening and satisfies most if not all of the screening principles described in Chapter 1. It is an important health problem—untreated it has serious consequences the most important of which is progressive mental retardation often with associated neurological damage. The mechanics of the condition are well understood (Komrower 1984). There is a suitable diagnostic test which is available, safe, and acceptable to the population. The Guthrie blood test (Guthrie and Susi 1963) is carried out routinely in the United Kingdom between the sixth and tenth day of life. The timing of the test is important because if it is done too early the evidence of impaired enzyme phenylalanine hydroxylase (PH) activity will not have had time to develop. It is a satisfactory and sensitive method. One-dimensional chromatography has also been widely used. It is equally sensitive but slightly more expensive although it can also detect increases in other amino-acids.

Phenylketonuria also satisfies the treatment principle and can be very effectively treated, essentially by diet. Although there is no firm evidence, it is generally agreed that a restricted phenylalanine intake should be continued as long as family and social conditions allow (Bickel 1980). Careful control of diet should certainly continue at least until 10 years of age (Komrower 1984).

Although more work on the cost-benefit aspect is needed, it seems reasonable to accept that screening for PKU can claim to be cost-effective. The prevention of severe mental retardation, apart from the human benefit, releases the community from providing expensive long-term medical and social supervision for an individual who is instead able to lead a normal and independent life (Komrower 1984).

That few people today have seen a case of untreated classical PKU in a young child is a testament to the success of the screening programme for this condition.

CONGENITAL HYPOTHYROIDISM

Congenital hypothyroidism (CH) is another condition which, untreated, can have devastating effects on a child's growth and development, both mental and physical. Neonatal screening is vital because, in most cases, the signs and symptoms of the condition develop after the neonatal period and clinical diagnosis is therefore likely to come too late to prevent damage (Panayotopoulos 1988). It is generally agreed that treatment should be started within six weeks of birth and that, if it is, intelligence in children with CH will be normal (Macfaul *et al* 1978). Initial analysis of the results of a collaborative European study suggests that even a short delay in starting treatment may affect outcome (Illig *et al* 1987). Thus, as with PKU, a congenital hypothyroidism is a prime candidate for screening in the neonatal period. The condition is reasonably well understood, and although it is relatively uncommon, its consequences for an untreated individual are appalling.

The screening procedure involves the collection of a blood spot on a filter paper (Guthrie card), although in a few cases screening is performed on umbilical cord serum (Illig *et al* 1982). There are two main approaches to the screening methodology and the choice of method remains the subject of debate. The first is to measure thyroid stimulating hormone (TSH) as the primary screening test and to regard raised TSH values as abnormal. The second is to measure thyroxine (T4) first, and if the values are below a certain level, to carry out a TSH test as well. The former is the approach used in most European countries including Britain, although there is variation even within one country. The main disadvantage of this method is that a small number of hypothyroid children will be missed if they are screened in the early neonatal period because of a delay in the development of the feedback regulation of pituitary TSH secretion. Both approaches, however, have their limitations, and it has been suggested that T4 measurement may discriminate better when the blood sample is taken around the third day of life and TSH when it is taken a few days later (Barnes 1985).

In the United States, screening of newborn babies for CH is mandatory in all stages (Stevens, Rigilano, and Wilson 1988; US Preventive Services Task Force 1989) and it was recommended also by the Canadian Task Force on the Periodic Health Examination (1979). Most European countries have national screening programmes for CH associated with those for PKU. In the United Kingdom, national screening for congenital hypothyroidism was established in 1982 (DHSS 1981) with a comprehensive programme covering over 99 per cent of live births and working with the established programme for PKU (MRC 1981). The United Kingdom screening programme uses mainly TSH measurement and the recommended age for screening is 6–14 days.

In a study which spanned the first three years of national screening, the incidence of CH in England, Wales and Northern Ireland was found to be 1 in just under 4000 births (Grant and Smith 1988). This agrees with estimates from elsewhere which produced a range of 1 in 3800–4000 infants worldwide (Fisher 1983). Four infants with primary hypothyroidism (0·8 per cent) were known to have been missed. Two of these—one in which a blood sample was not taken and one false-negative result—might have been prevented. The other two had defects of thyroxine synthesis and showed normal concentrations of TSH at screening. However, over a quarter of infants detected as having CH by screening using measurement of TSH had plasma thyroxine levels within the normal range (Grant and Smith 1988). The small number of missed cases suggest that fewer false-negative results will arise with measurements of TSH than T4 and that the benefits of a second screening test would be small. However, T4 measurement can detect the rare cases of secondary or tertiary CH which are not suspected clinically and which TSH screening alone will not identify (Layde 1984).

Results of a retrospective study in Sweden (Alm *et al* 1984) indicated that CH will be underdiagnosed if clinical signs and symptoms are used as indicators and that those diagnosed in this way will be detected too late to prevent damage. Screening is recommended although this may result in a degree of overdiagnosis and overtreatment. In the United Kingdom study (Grant and Smith, 1988), this possibility was recognised and a letter was sent to paediatricians soon after the start of screening in which the need to withdraw treatment temporarily at some time after the age of 1 year was emphasised, particularly in children with no clinical features of hypothyroidism or in whom thyroid function was borderline at diagnosis. The authors comment that 'the records of the register suggest that this advice was heeded only to a limited extent'.

The cost of screening for congenital hypothyroidism,

especially in conjunction with PKU, is relatively low and its cost-effectiveness has been documented (Layde *et al* 1979, Layde 1984). The costs are those of collecting the blood samples, analysing with in the laboratory, and treating those diagnosed. The benefits are the averted costs of the long-term care of untreated cases and the improved productivity of the CH infant treated early. An economic analysis of CH screening in the United States in the late 1970s (Layde *et al* 1979), using a discount rate of 7·5 per cent estimated that the cost of detecting a case of CH by screening and of treating that case was around $11,800. The current value of the economic benefits of early treatment was estimated at $105,000 per case, giving a cost-benefit ratio of about 1:9.

Screening for congenital hypothyroidism is another relative success story. But there remain variations between different parts of the United Kingdom both in methods and cut-off levels used, standardisation, and quality control.

CONGENITAL DISLOCATION OF THE HIP

Neonatal screening for congenital dislocation of the hip (CDH)—one of the most common congenital defects of the locomotor system—still excites a great deal of debate.

Frankenburg (1981) suggested that it is unethical to screen for CDH because it is unethical to mount a large scale screening programme unless one can assure a benefit. He reminds us of the three questions, set by Illingworth in 1971, for assessing the ethics of any clinical investigations: what good may it do? what harm may it do? what harm may be done by not doing it?.

Cunningham and colleagues (1984) asked whether the frequency of treatable abnormalities in the hips would justify clinical and radiological examination of all 4 month old infants in the neonatal period? They claimed their experience showed that it would—5·5 per cent of the children in their population with minor signs had abnormalities requiring further supervision.

Roberton (1984) strongly disagreed with this on three grounds. Firstly, most hips which are unstable in the first few days of life recover spontaneously. Secondly, 25–50 per cent of dislocated and dislocatable hips present in infancy, having been missed at neonatal examination. Thirdly, the need for surgery in CDH has not changed in last 30 years. Roberton concludes that either the incidence of CDH is increasing or our screening efforts have been a complete failure.

Knox, Armstrong and Lancashire (1987) looked at the incidence of CDH in Birmingham in three time sectors—1942–52, 1950–54, and 1974–83. Despite the introduction of neonatal screening for CDH in Birmingham in late 1966, they found no evidence that CDH requiring prolonged treatment had declined. The performance of the screening procedure was poor—it detected only a third of genuine dislocations, and false positives outnumbered true positives by a ratio of 10:1. Since failures were particularly associated with hospitals where the clinical services were well organised, Knox and colleagues suggest that one of the problems may be a faulty understanding of the natural history of this condition.

Leck (1986) summarised four main problem areas in screening for this condition as currently practised. The first concerns false-positive results. Most of the screened cases in which unstable hips are reported are false positives at least in the sense that they would not progress to dislocation if untreated. Although it is widely believed that these cases are pre-disposed to osteoarthrosis which may be reduced by treating the instability in the neonatal period, this has not been examined in epidemiological studies. It is, therefore, at least possible that several infants suffer unnecessary treatment for every one who benefits. This danger of overtreatment was examined also in a study of twins in Norway (Kramer, Berg, and Nance 1987). Their results also suggest that neonatal screening programmes may have low specificity in detecting cases that require treatment and recommend that the efficacy of screening for this condition should be carefully examined. It may be that the development of ultrasound screening may help to improve diagnosis of CDH and reduce over-treatment (Berman and Klenerman 1986).

The second problem is false-negative results. The prevalence of false negatives in which a hip that appeared stable when screened but is later reported to be dislocated varies widely in screened populations but seems to be of about the same order as the number of true positives. It is not known how often in these false-negative cases instability is present but missed in neonatal screening and how often it develops later.

The third problem area identified by Leck (1986) concerns treatment policies where at least three questions are still disputed by experts—should the indications for treatment include abnormal physical signs short of actual dislocation and dislocatability; should treatment be started immediately or postponed to see if signs persist; and what type of splint should be used?

Fourthly, there is considerable doubt about the outcome of early treatment. In a study on 23,002 children in Bristol—a recognised centre of excellence in this field—screening appeared to do no more than halve the frequency of established dislocation of the hip and had negligible effects on health care costs (Dunn *et al* 1983). It has also been suggested, that one of the manipulations involved in the screening procedure may be potentially harmful and may actually create instability in some hip joints (Cheetham *et al* 1983; Leck 1986). Cheetham and colleagues (1983) strongly deprecate the widespread use of Barlow's test by inexperienced personnel in the first 48 hours of life and 'deplore the growing tendency to abandon splinting newborn dislocated hips until there is more evidence that it does harm'. They suggest that a small team of experienced professionals with a long-term commitment are best able to diagnose cases without causing damage to hips at a vulnerable time. There have been reports (for example, Mackenzie and Wilson 1981, Cunningham *et al* 1984) of screened populations in which the reported prevalence of late diagnosed cases of cases of hip dislocation exceeded the overall prevalence in unscreened populations. And the report of one screening study showed that the incidence of dislocation had trebled since the introduction of screening (Catford *et al* 1982).

Bartsocas (1988), in a recent review of the subject, suggests that formal screening for CDH should not be included in neonatal screening programmes. He advocates instead a thorough physical examination soon after birth and again on follow-up at 4 to 6 weeks together with efforts to increase awareness of the problem in health professionals and parents and special training in examination techniques where appropriate for the former.

However, screening for CDH has also been studied in detail recently by an expert working party in the United Kingdom (DHSS 1986). The incidence of unstable hips in the neonatal period is about 15–20 per 1000 but only 10 per cent of these will become dislocated and a further 10 per cent may show evidence of subluxation or dysplasia. The early detection of the condition is thought to be worthwhile because response to treatment is likely to be better if it starts before the age of weight-bearing (Dwyer 1987). Dwyer also emphasises the absolute necessity of having proper intensive training on examination techniques as the screening procedure is often entrusted to relatively junior staff. Newer diagnostic aids, such as electronic augmentation for interpretation of clinical signs and ultrasound scanning, should improve the position. Leck (1986) also makes the point that at this stage treatment will have less impact on the physical and psychosocial development of the infant and on family life.

The DHSS working group recognised the difficulties and pitfalls of screening for this condition but recommended that screening in the form of regular examinations should continue. The possibility of CDH should be considered whenever a child is seen in the first two years of life—a single neonatal examination will miss cases which develop later. Their specific recommendations were that a child should have an examination for CDH at the following times: within 24 hours of birth; on discharge from hospital or within 10 days of birth; at 6 weeks of age; at 6–9 months; at 15–21 months. Gait should be reviewed at 24–30 months and again at pre-school or school entry. The Ortolani/Barlow manoeuvre can be used for the first three examinations but is not appropriate after the age of 3 months.

Hall and colleagues (1989) made four comments on the DHSS report. Firstly, they emphasised that much remains to be learned about the natural history of CDH and there is particular concern about the poor specificity and sensitivity of the neonatal examination. Secondly, because of the increasing trend towards early discharge from hospital after birth, it may be more difficult to ensure that the second check is carried out. They suggest that the yield of new cases from this examination should be determined and if it is such as to justify this particular recommendation, existing arrangements will have to be re-assessed and improved. Thirdly, the examination at 15–21 months does not coincide with any other examinations currently recommended and a more realistic time scale might be between 18 and 24 months. Fourthly, children with neurological disease, especially spastic cerebral palsy, are at high risk of CDH throughout childhood and should be under specialist supervision.

They recommend continuation of the screening programme for congenital dislocation of the hip but stress the need for further monitoring of the yield of the expanded programme recommended in the DHSS working party report.

Considerable uncertainty on the value of screening for this condition clearly exists. The existing test procedures are unsatisfactory in a number of ways, standards of expertise are very variable, and there is a disturbing lack of evaluation. Leck (1986) suggested that randomised clinical trials should be set up to enable the costs and benefits of current neontal screening policies to be compared with those of screening later in infancy and of not screening but treating CDH when it presents clinically. 'Whether screening is justified,' he states, 'will remain an open question until this is done.'

DEVELOPMENTAL DISORDERS

In an answer to a parliamentary question about national screening priorities in June 1989, the Minister for Health in Scotland stated that

> following birth, children are screened for inherited or developmental conditions and this is continued throughout the school years.

Hall and colleagues (1989) define developmental screening as

> the performance of one or more developmental examination on every child at specified key ages in infancy... As with other screening tests, the aim is to examine all apparently normal children in order to identify those who may have some undetected abnormality.

They concluded that there is no justification for this type of repeated routine screening examination for all infants and children as a means of diagnosing serious disorders and impairments and included the following clear recommendations on screening in this area.

1. No programme for detection of these conditions can fulfil the screening criteria.

2. Early detection is worthwhile.

3. The main means of detection are health service response to parental concern, competent follow-up of high-risk cases, neonatal examination for recognition of syndromes, and easy access to professional expertise.

They also stressed the need for health surveillance as a vital framework for early detection and for health professionals to have a thorough knowledge of child development to enable them to evaluate the significance of parental concerns. With these provisos they suggest that routine developmental screening can safely be discontinued, with the advantage that this should release more professional time to devote to those parents and children who need expert help and support but at present do not always receive it.

This is one of the aspects of the Hall Report that has caused the most controversy. As Wilson (1990) has pointed out, much routine repeated developmental screening is probably unnecessary in that experienced practitioners will identify abnormal development by listening to parents, taking competent histories, and observing children at play. However he stresses that the less experienced and trainees will still learn best by using developmental check lists.

Bax and Whitmore (1990), who are strongly critical of the Hall Report, rightly also drew attention to the intractable problem of at-risk families who may escape the health care net altogether—single parent families, those in inner city areas of high deprivation, travelling people, immigrant families from very different cultures. Reliance on parental concern about a child's development pre-supposes firstly the existence of that concern and secondly the opportunity and ability to express it.

We would suggest that it might be prudent to make any changes in developmental testing the subject of trials in one or two areas in the first instance to see, for example, whether resources released by the cessation of repeated developmental testing could be used to identify and help those most at risk.

SUMMARY

In the neonatal period we suggest that there is a continuing need for routine opportunistic screening of babies within the normal framework of health care already provided by good general practice teams. Screening for phenylketonuria and congenital hypothyroidism, which can be done in conjunction with each other, is beneficial and well established and should be routine. The evidence on screening for congenital dislocation of the hip seems much less conclusive and there is clearly a need for trials to evaluate the current policy of routine neonatal screening in comparison with the options of screening later in infancy or not screening at all but treating CDH when it presents clinically. Resources currently devoted to the repeated routine developmental screening of all babies might be more usefully concentrated on those in need of special care. However, as suggested earlier, it may be wise to monitor the effect of such a change of policy in specified areas to see whether those considered to be most at risk can be reached and do benefit from increased attention.

CONCLUSIONS

During the 1970s there was a great deal of discussion about the possibilities for prevention through antenatal and neonatal screening. There has been progress but, as with so much of screening, applications and standards vary in different parts of the country, responsibility remains fragmented, and there is an urgent need for greater integration and clarification of professional responsibility and quality control, and for more emphasis on screening for prevention.

Wald (1984) has suggested that responsibility for screening services should be concentrated on one department—possibly the Department of Community or Preventive or Public Health Medicine. He wrote

> One of the challenges of the next decade will be to organise health services so that screening programmes are well chosen and effectively applied in the community.

We are now six years into the decade to which Wald refers and the position remains extremely patchy. One major advance, discussed elsewhere in this book, would be the appointment of a senior person with responsibility for screening in every Health Authority area. It is also important to reiterate that screening for a particular disorder or group of conditions should not be continued simply because it has always been done. The Hall Report is a good example of the critical approach that we need to adopt on all aspects of screening before we can claim to be beginning to provide an acceptable service.

REFERENCES

ALES, K. L. AND SANTINI, D. L. 'Should all pregnant women be screened for gestational glucose intolerance?' *Lancet* 1989, 1:1187–91.

ALM, J., HAGENFELDT, L., LARSSON, A. AND LUNDBERG, K. 'Incidence of congenital hypothyroidism: retrospective study of neonatal laboratory screening versus clinical symptoms as indicators leading to diagnosis. *Br Med J* 1984, 289:1171–5.

BARNES, N. D. 'Screening for congenital hypothyroidism: the first decade'. *Arch Dis Child* 1985, 60:587–92.

BARTSOCAS, C. 'Congenital hip dislocation'. In *Elimination or Reduction of Diseases*. SILMAN, A. J. AND ALLWRIGHT, SHANE P. A. (eds). Oxford: Oxford University Press, 1988.

BAX, M. C. O. AND WHITMORE, K. 'Health for all children'. (Book review). *Arch Dis Child* 1990, 65:141–2.

BERMAN, L. AND KLENERMAN, L. 'Ultrasound screening for hip abnormalities: preliminary findings in 1001 neonates'. *Br Med J* 1986, 293:719–22.

BICKEL, J. *Phenylketonuria, past, present, future.* (F. P. Hudson Memorial Lecture, Leeds 1979). H. Inherit Metab Dis 1980,3:123.

CAMPBELL-BROWN, M., McFADYEN, I. R., SEAL, D. V. AND STEPHENSON, M. L. 'Is screening for bacteriuria in pregnancy worth while? *Br Med J* 1987, 294:1579–82.

'Canadian Task Force on the Periodic Health Examination. The periodic health examination'. *Can Med Assoc J* 1979, 121:1–45.

CARSTAIRS, V. AND COLE, S. 'Spina bifida and anencephaly in Scotland'. *Br Med J* 1984:289:1182–4.

CATFORD, J. C., BENNET, G. C., AND WILKINSON, J. A. 'Congenital hip dislocation: an increasing and still uncontrolled disability? *Br Med J* 1982, 285:1527–30.

CENTERS FOR DISEASE CONTROL. 'Public health guidelines for enhancing diabetes control through maternal and child health programs.' *Morbid Mortal Weekly Rep* 1986, 35:201–13.

CHAMBERLAIN, J. 'The benefits and costs of prenatal diagnosis' (editorial). *Rev Epidemiol Sante Publique* 1984, 32:85–7.

CHAPPLE, J. Personal communication, 1990.

CHEETHAM, C. H., GARROW, D. H., TARIN, P. and MEDHURST, A. W. J. 'Congenital dislocation of the hip'. *Br Med J* 1983, 286:227.

COMMITTEE ON OBSTETRICS: 'Maternal and Fetal Medicine'. Newsletter. Washington DC. American College of Obstetricians and Gynecologists. January 1987:9.

CRANDALL, B. F., HOWARD, J., LEBHERZ, T. B., RUBINSTEIN, L., SAMPLE, W. F. AND SARN, D. 'Follow-up of 2000 second trimester amniocenteses'. *Obst Gynecol* 1980, 56:625–8.

CUCKLE, H. S. AND WALD, N. J. 'Principles of screening'. In *Antenatal and Neonatal Screening*. N. J. WALD (ed.). Oxford: Oxford University Press, 1984.

CUCKLE, H. S. AND WALD, N. J. 'Screening for Down Syndrome'. In *Prenatal Diagnosis*. R. J. LILFORD (ed.). London: Butterworths, 1990.

CUNNINGHAM, K. T., MOULTON, A., BENINGFIELD, S. A. AND MADDOCK, C. R. 'A clicking hip in a newborn baby should never be ignored'. *Lancet* 1984 1:668–70.

DAVIES, B. AND DORAN,T. 'Factors in a woman's decision to undergo gentic amniocentesis for advanced maternal age? *Nurs Res* 1982, 31:56–9.

DEPARTMENT OF HEALTH AND SOCIAL SECURITY. *Screening for early detection of Congenital Hypothyroidism.* London: HMSO, 1981.

DEPARTMENT OF HEALTH AND SOCIAL SECURITY. *Screening for the detection of congenital dislocation of the hip.* London: HMSO, 1986.

DOLL, SIR RICHARD. Foreword. In *Antenatal and Neonatal Screening*. N. J. WALD (ed.). Oxford: Oxford University Press, 1984.

DRILLIEN, C. M. AND WILKINSON, E. M. 'Mongolism: when should parents be told? *Br Med J* 1964, 2:1306–7.

DUNN, P. M., EVANS, R. E., GRIFFITHS, H., WITHEROW, P. J. 'Congenital dislocation of the hip: the preliminary results of a 10 year screening programme in Bristol 1970–79'. *Arch Dis Child* 1983, 58:654–5.

DWYER, N ST J. P. 'Congenital dislocation of the hip: to screen or not to screen. *Arch Dis Child* 1987, 62:635–7.

ELIAS, S. AND ANNAS, G. J. 'Routine prenatal genetic screening'. *N Engl J Med* 1987, 317:1407–8.

ELWOOD, J. M. AND ELWOOD, J. H. *Epidemiology of anencephaly and spina bifida.* Oxford: Oxford University Press, 1980.

EUROCAT. *Surveillance of congenital anomalies. Years 1980–1983. An EEC concerted action project.* Brussels, 1986.

EVERETT, W. D. 'Screening for gestational diabetes: an analysis of health benefits and costs.' *Am J Prev Med* 1989, 1:38–43.

FEARN, J., HIBBARD, B. M. AND ROBINSON, J. O. 'Screening for neural-tube defects and maternal anxiety' *Br J Obstet Gynaecol* 1982, 89:218–21.

FISHER, D. A. Second International Conference on Neonatal Thyroid Screening: progress report. *J Pediat* 1983, 102:653–4.

FRANKENBURG, W. H. 'To screen or not to screen: congenital dislocation of the hip'. *Am J Publ Hlth* 1981, 71:1311–13.

GILL, O. N., ADLER, M. W. AND DAY, N. E. 'Monitoring the prevalence of HIV. Foundations for a programme of unlinked anonymous testing in England and Wales'. *Br Med J* 1989, 299:1295–98.

GILLON, R. 'Testing for HIV without permission'. *Br Med J* 1987, 294:821–23.

GOUJARD, J. 'Down syndrome and neural tube defects'. In *Elimination or Reduction of Diseases*. A. J. SILMAN, AND SHANE P. A. ALLWRIGHT (eds). Oxford: Oxford University Press, 1988.

GRANT, D. B. AND SMITH, I. 'Survey of neonatal screening for primary hypothyroidism in England, Wales, and Northern Ireland 1982–4.' *Br Med J* 1988, 296:1355–8.

GUTHRIE, R. AND SUSI, A. 'A simple phenylalanine method for the detection of phenylketonuria in large populations of newborn infants'. *Pediatrics* 1963, 32:338–43.

HALL, D. M. B. (ed.) *Health for All Children. Report of the Joint Working Party on Child Health Surveillance*. Oxford: Oxford University Press, 1989.

HERINGA, M. AND HUISJES, H. J. 'Prenatal screening: current policy in EC countries'. *Eur J Obstet Gynecol Reprod Biol* 1988, 28 (Suppl): 7–52.

HIBBARD, B. M., ROBERTS, C. J., ELDER, G. H., EVANS, K. T. AND LAURENCE, K. M. 'Can we afford screening for neural tube defects? The South Wales experience'. *Br Med J* 1985, 290:293–5.

HOLLAND, W. W. 'Screening for Disease. Taking stock'. *Lancet* 1974, ii:1494–7.

ILLIG, R., LARGO, R. H., QIN, Q., TORRESANI, T., ROCHICCIOLI, P. AND LARSSON, A. 'Mental development in congenital hypothyroidism after neonatal screening'. *Arch Dis child* 1987, 62:1050–5.

ILLIG, R., LARSSON, A. AND ROCHICCIOLI, P. *Report on the European Society for Pediatric Endocrinology Collaborative Study on Congenital Hypothyroidism*. 21st Annual meeting of the ESPE, Helsinki, 1982.

ILLINGWORTH, R. S. 'Discussion of diagnostic catheter examinations of the newborn by Norman T. Quinn'. *Clin Pediatr* 1971, 10:254.

JARRETT, R. J. 'Diabetes mellitus and gestational diabetes'. In *Antenatal and Neonatal Screening*. N. J. WALD (ed.). Oxford: Oxford University Press, 1984.

KNOX, E. G., ARMSTRONG, E. H., AND LANCASHIRE, R. J. 'Effectiveness of screening for congenital dislocation of the hip'. *J Epid Comm Hlth* 1987, 41:282–9.

KOMROWER, G. M. 'Phenylketonuria and other inherited metabolic defects'. In *Antenatal and Neonatal Screening*. N. J. WALD (ed.). Oxford: Oxford University Press, 1984.

KRAMER, A. A., BERG, K. AND NANCE, W. E. 'The effect of perinatal screening in Norway on the magnitude of noninherited risk factors for congenital dislocation of the hip'. *Am J Epid* 1987, 125:271–6.

KULIEV, A. M. 'The WHO Control program for Hereditary Anemias'. Birth Defects Original Article Series, 23 (5B), 383–394. March of Dimes Birth Defects Foundation, 1988.

LAYDE, P. M. 'Congenital hypothyroidism'. In *Antenatal and Neonatal Screening*. N. J. WALD (ed.). Oxford: Oxford University Press, 1984.

LAYDE, P. M., VON ALLMEN, S. D. AND OAKLEY, G. P. 'Congenital hypothyroidism control programs. A cost-benefit analysis'. *JAMA* 1979, 241:2290–2.

LECK, I. 'An epidemiological assessment of neonatal screening for dislocation of the hip'. *J R Coll Phys (Lond)* 1986, 20:56–62.

MACFAUL, R., DORNER, S., BRETT, E. M. AND GRANT, D. B. 'Neurological abnormalities in patients treated for hypothyroidism from early life'. *Arch Dis Child* 1978, 53:611–19.

MACINTYRE, S. *'Expectations and experiences of first pregnancy.* Aberdeen: MRC Medical Sociology Unit, 1981.

MACKENZIE, I. G. AND WILSON, J. G. 'Problems encountered in the early diagnosis and management of congenital dislocation of the hip'. *J Bone Jt Surg* 1981, 63 B:38–42.

MARTEAU, T. M., KIDD, J., COOK, R., JOHNSTON, M., MICHIE, S., SHAW, R. W. AND SLACK, J. Screening for Down's syndrome. *Br Med J* 1988, 297, 1469.

MATTHEWS, R. N. *Monitoring progress in thalassaemia major: what is important for the patient?* Birth Defects: Original Article Series, 1988, 23 (5B), 227–32.

MEDICAL RESEARCH COUNCIL OF CANADA. *Diagnosis of genetic disease by amniocentesis during the second trimester of pregnancy.* A Canadian Study. Report No 5. Canada: Supply Services, 1977.

MEDICAL RESEARCH COUNCIL STEERING COMMITTEE FOR THE MRC/DHSS PHENYLKETONURIA REGISTER. Routine neonatal screening for phenylketonuria in the United Kingdom 1964–78'. *Br Med J* 1981, 282:1680–4.

MEDICAL RESEARCH COUNCIL. 'Working Party on Amniocentesis: an assessment of the hazards of amniocentesis. *Br J Obstet Gyaecol* 1978, 85 (suppl 2):1–4.

MENNUTI, M. T. 'Prenatal diagnosis—advances bring new challenges'. (Editorial). *N Engl J Med* 1989, 320:661–3.

MILNE, R. I. G. 'Assessment of care of children with sickle cell disease: implications for neonatal screening programmes'. *Br Med J* 1990, 300:371–4.

MODELL, B. AND PETROU, M. 'Review of Control Programs and Future Trends in the United Kingdom'. *Eur J Obstet Gynecol Reprod Biol* 1988, 28 (Suppl):433–42.

70   ANTENATAL AND NEONATAL SCREENING

MODELL, B. PETROU, M., WARD, T. H. T., FAIRWEATHER, D. V. I., RODECK, C., VARNAVIDES, L. A. AND WHITE, J. M. 'Effect of fetal diagnostic testing on birth-rate of thalassaemia major in Britain'. *Lancet* 1984, 3:1383-6.

MODELL, B., WARD, R. H. T. and FAIRWEATHER, D. V. I. 'Effect of introducing antenatal diagnosis on reproductive behaviour of families at risk for thalassaemia major'. *Br Med J* 1980, 280:1347-50.

MORRELL, DAVID. Personal communication, 1990.

MUIR GRAY, J. A. 'Needs of the Community'. In *Antenatal and Neonatal Screening*. N. J. WALD (ed.). Oxford: Oxford University Press, 1984.

NATIONAL INSTITUTE FOR CHILD HEALTH AND DEVELOPMENT. 'National Registry for for amniocentesis study group. Mid-trimester amniocentesis for prenatal diagnosis. Safety and accuracy'. *JAMA* 1976, 236:1471-6.

NIELSON, C. 'An encounter with modern medical technology: women's experiences with amniocentesis'. *Women Health* 1981, 6:109-24.

OFFICE OF POPULATION CENSUSES AND SURVEYS. *Congenital malformation statistics, 1971-80*. London: HMSO, 1983.

OLD, J. M., WARD, R. H. T., PETROU, M., KARAGOZLOU, F., MODELL, B., WEATHERALL, D. J. *'First trimester fetal diagnosis for haemoglobinopathies: three cases'*. *Lancet* 1982, 2:1413-6.

PANAYOTOPOULOS, T. 'Congenital hypothyroidism'. In *Elimination or Reduction of Diseases*. A. J. SILMAN AND SHANE P. A. ALLWRIGHT (eds). Oxford: Oxford University Press, 1988.

PETRIDOU, E. AND LOUKOPOULOS, D. 'THALASSAEMIA' in *Elimination or Reduction of Diseases*. A. J. SILMAN, AND SHANE P. ALLWRIGHT (Eds). Oxford: Oxford University Press, 1988.

REID, MARGARET. 'Consumer-oriented studies in relation to prenatal screening tests. *Eur J Obstet Gynecol Reprod Biol* 1988, 28 (Suppl): 79-92.

'Report of the UK Collaborative Study on Alpha-fetoprotein in relation to Neural Tube Defects. Maternal serum alpha-fetoprotein measurement in antenatal screening for anencephaly and spina bifida in early pregnancy'. *Lancet* 1977, 1:1323-32.

RHOADS, G. G., JACKSON, L. G., SCHLESSELMAN, S. E. *et al*. 'The safety and efficiency of chorionic villus sampling for early prenatal diagnosis of cytogenetic abnormalities'. *N Engl J Med* 1989, 320:609-17.

ROBERTON, N. C. R. 'Screening for congenital dislocation of the hip'. *Lancet* 1984, 1:909-10.

ROBINSON, J. O., HIBBARD, B. M. AND LAURENCE, K. M. 'Anxiety during a crisis: emotional effects of screening for neural tube defects'. *J. Psychosom Res* 1984, 28:163-9.

SCHMIDT, E. 'Distribution of health personnel and neonatal care'. In

Perinatal Care Delivery Systems: Description and Evaluation in European Community Countries. M. KAMINSKI, G. BREART, P. BUEKENS, H. J. HUISJES, G. MCILWAINE, AND H.-K. SELBMANN, (eds). Oxford: Oxford University Press, 1986.

STEVENS, M. B., RIGILANO, J. C. AND WILSON, C. C. 'State screening for metabolic disorders in newborns'. *Am Fam Physician* 1988, 37:223–8.

STONE, DAVID H., SMALLS, MARY J., ROSENBERG, KATHRYN, AND WOMERSLEY, JOHN. 'Screening for congenital neural tube defects in a high-risk area: an epidemiological perspective.' *J Epidemiol Comm Hlth* 1988, 42:271–3.

STONE, DAVID H., ROSENBERG, KATHRYN, AND WOMERSLEY, JOHN. 'Recent trends in the prevalence and secondary prevention of Down's syndrome'. *Paed Perinat Epidemiol* 1989, 3:278–83.

TABOR, A., MADSEN, M., OBEL, E. B., PHILIP, J., BANG, J., AND NOGAARD-PEDERSEN, B. Randomised controlled trial of genetic amniocentesis in 4606 low-risk women'. *Lancet* 1986, 1:1287–93.

TABOR, A., PHILIP, J., BANG, J., MADSEN, M, OBEL, E. B., NOGAARD-PEDERSEN, B. 'Needle size and risk of miscarriage after amniocentesis'. *Lancet* 1988, 1:183–4.

UK Collaborative Study on alpha-fetoprotein in relation to neural tube defects. First Report. 'Maternal serum alpha-fetoprotein measurement in antenatal screening for anencephaly and spina bifida in early pregnancy'. *Lancet* 1977, 1:1323–32.

US PREVENTIVE SERVICES TASK FORCE. *Guide to Clinical Preventive Services.* Baltimore: Williams and Wilkins, 1989.

WALD, N. J. 'Conclusions'. In *Antenatal and Neonatal Screening.* N. J. WALD (ed.). Oxford: Oxford University Press, 1984.

WALD, N. J. AND CUCKLE, H. S. 'Open neural tube defects'. In *Antenatal and Neonatal Screening.* N. J. WALD (ed.). Oxford: Oxford University Press, 1984.

WALD, N. J., CUCKLE, H. S., DENSEM, J. W., NANCHALHAL, K., ROYSTON, P., CHARD, T., HADDOW, J. E., KNIGHT, G. J., PALOMAKI, G. E. AND CANICK, J. A. 'Maternal serum screening for Down's syndrome in early pregnancy'. *Br Med J* 1988, 297:883–7.

WALD, N. J., TERZIAN, E., VICKERS, P. A. AND WEATHERALL, J. A. C. 'Congenital talipes and hip malformation in relation to amniocentesis: a case control study'. *Lancet* 1983, 2:246–9.

WEATHERALL, D. J., OLD, J. M., THEIN, S. L., WAINSCOAT, J. S. AND CLEGG, J. B. 'Prenatal diagnosis of the common haemoglobin disorders'. *J Med Genet*, 1985, 22:422–30.

WILSON, J. A. *Health for all children.* (Book review). *Arch Dis Child* 1990, 65:142.

WORLD HEALTH ORGANIZATION WORKING GROUP. 'Hereditary anaemias: genetic basis, clinical features, diagnosis and treatment'. *Bull* WHO 1982, 60:643–60.

3 SCREENING AND SURVEILLANCE IN CHILDHOOD

Childhood: the period of human life
interned between the idiocy of infancy and
the folly of youth.
(AMBROSE BIERCE: *The Devil's Dictionary*)

INTRODUCTION

SCREENING AND SURVEILLANCE IN CHILDHOOD,
—defined for our purposes as age 1–11 years—are
extremely important. Theoretically at least, this should
be the time to build on the relationship between health
professionals and parents established at the antenatal
and neonatal stages, to encourage sensible habits in
relation to the child's health, and to detect abnormalities or disorders at an early stage when effective
treatment or intervention is available. There is also the
potential for preventing the foundations of future ill
health from being laid. Holland and Reid (1965) and
Barker and Osmond (1986), for example, have drawn
attention to evidence suggesting a causal connection
between acute lower respiratory infection in childhood
and chronic bronchitis later in life. Thus a high uptake
of immunisation for measles with its major complication
risk of pneumonia, will not only have a beneficial effect
on mortality and morbidity in childhood but is likely to
reduce the incidence of chronic bronchitis in adults. It
is also true that, since the main cause of death in those
aged under 14 in England and Wales is accidents—
apart from congenital anomalies in the 1–4 year age
group—a satisfactory level of health service contact
with the parents and with the children themselves
through a good system of screening and surveillance

72

should provide opportunities for advice and education on various aspects of home and road safety.

The Royal College of General Practitioners Joint Working Party on Child Health Surveillance (Hall 1989) has recently provided a welcome review of child health surveillance, mentioned in the previous chapter, and we will consider its findings and recommendations here. There is in general practice, in child health clinics, and in the school health service a long-established tradition of child health surveillance and screening in the United Kingdom. However, this tradition brings into sharp relief many of the problems associated with screening in general that are perhaps most clearly illustrated in this sector of the life-cycle. These can be broadly divided into four categories: differing definitions; involvement of various groups of health professionals leading to confusion and duplication; variation of provision and standard of service in different areas of the country; paucity of proper scientific evaluation of results of screening. We will consider these categories briefly here and return to them later in the book.

DEFINITIONS

The definitions of surveillance, screening, and assessment in relation to developmental screening for pre-school children have been recently summarised by Bain (1989). Surveillance is a continuing process throughout childhood and is part of the normal contact general practitioners would expect to have with the children on their lists. Screening is a specific contact made by a health-worker with an apparently healthy child to try to identify any mental or physical disorder, defects of sight or hearing and so on. Assessment is a more specialised examination because of identification of a suspected abnormality or presence of particular risk factors.

Bain (1989) examines the advantages and disadvantages of screening in primary care. The former might include the building of a more positive relationship between the doctor and health visitor and the children and their parents, opportunities for advice on minor problems which would not normally be brought to medical attention, improved immunisation rates, and early diagnosis of conditions which can be identified and dealt with. Disadvantages would include amount of time and resources expended on routine examination of normal children, and differential attendance at clinics, with non-attendance highest in the lower socio-economic groups at highest risk of illness.

In a critical review of child health surveillance in primary care, Butler (1989) offers a further set of definitions. He uses the term surveillance exclusively to mean secondary prevention. This can be subdivided into individual surveillance and population surveillance, and the former can be further subdivided into screening, case-finding, and non-specific oversight. He notes with justification that 'no set of definitions can be produced that will harmonise with the entire body of literature on preventive child health care'.

In the Hall report (1989), surveillance is defined in its broadest sense to cover assessment and monitoring of the physical, social, and emotional health and development of all children, offering and arranging appropriate intervention when necessary, preventing disease by immunisation and other means, and health education.

One criticism that has been made of the Working Party's approach is that they have judged surveillance activities using prescriptive screening criteria.

> Most medical activity is not encompassed in these very strict criteria and the working party give no reasons why they should be applied to the task of child health surveillance
> (Bax and Whitmore, 1990).

Surveillance may be important in identifying disabilities and problems, both clinically and epidemiologically, for example in relation to suitable educational placement, while failing completely to alter the natural history of specific disorders, such as speech defects or neuromotor impairments.

There thus remains confusion and controversy on the use of the terms surveillance and screening in child health and we would contend that a rigid distinction between them is unrealistic in practice. In the present climate, where health promotion and prevention of illness are becoming an integral part of health care, particularly at primary care level, we would see screening in childhood as a specific tool of the more general programme of health surveillance to be used for particular conditions or in particular high-risk groups.

WHO DOES WHAT?

Responsibility for the health care of children in the United Kingdom currently lies with various types of health professionals—general practitioners and related health professionals including health visitors, community paediatricians, clinical medical officers, and in some instances hospital doctors and staff, are involved. There should also be increasing and regular involvement of dentists and optometrists, and an important source of practical advice can also be the pharmacist in the local chemist's shop. These opportunities for health service contact in childhood are summarised in Table 9.

TABLE 9. *Opportunities for health service contact in childhood*

LOCATION	TYPE OF HEALTH PROFESSIONAL
General practice	GP, health visitor, practice nurse
Hospital	Paediatrician, other specialist medical or paramedical hospital staff as appropriate
School	Clinical medical officer, school nurse, dentist, educational psychologist, speech therapist
Community	Clinical medical officer, dentist, optometrist, pharmacist

This multiplicity of involvement can lead to confusion and duplication if communication between professionals and services is not effective (Royal College of General Practitioners 1982). It is also likely that some children—usually those at greatest risk—may escape the health net altogether. Among the recommendations of the Hall Report (1989) is that primary health care teams should assume responsibility for ensuring that all children are seen at the appropriate ages. They also recommend that one individual in each District or Health Board should assume responsibity for overseeing the programme of surveillance.

The role of parents, often neglected in the past, is of increasing importance in this area. Involved and informed parents provide probably the best, and most cost-effective, system of quality and co-ordination control available, and this is being increasingly recognised. As the Hall Report (1989) states

> Surveillance, like other aspects of health care, has to be sensitive to the views of the consumer. Parents expect to be consulted about decisions that involve their children and increasingly are prepared to challenge professional expertise and advice.

The report lays particular emphasis on the important role of parents both in detecting and in acknowledging the possibility of developmental problems. Once again, however, this does not solve the problem of how to reach the minority of children most at risk whose parents cannot be relied on to notice let alone express concern about health or development.

In this context, Waller and Morgan (1988) draw attention to the fact that in the United Kingdom, despite increasing emphasis on the role of prevention in health care, participation in any schemes of health screening and surveillance has always remained a voluntary activity. There is no compulsion on parents to bring their children for developmental checks, for example, or to receive immunisation. This contrasts with the position in the United States where school entry is

dependent on immunisation. Parents carry some responsibility for the poor uptake in Britain but a *Lancet*
editorial (1987) suggests that professional disorganisa-
tion and lack of commitment may be more important
than social factors and leads to wide variation in
different Health Authority areas. This is well illustrated
by the fact that uptake of measles immunisation in 1985
in Blackpool District was 49·6 per cent whereas in
Macclesfield it was 91 per cent (DHSS 1986). In France
where statutory medical examinations of children are
carried out at certain specified ages, failure to comply
can result in witholding of child allowance (Royal
College of General Practitioners 1983).

In 1977 the World Health Organisation set a target of
90 per cent primary immunisation for all children under
2 years by 1990 (Begg and Noah 1985). There are three
main sources of immunisation—the general practitioner, child health clinics, and schools but provision is
very varied and unco-ordinated. As Jarman and colleagues (1988) have shown the average uptake of
measles immunisation from DHSS data for 191 District
Health Authorities for 1983–85 was 69 per cent. For 60
Districts, however, uptake was below 65 per cent and
for 15 below 50 per cent. The situation with regard to
immunisation in Britain at the moment is, therefore, far
from satisfactory and there are those who feel that some
form of compulsion should be considered. A less
dramatic form of action would be to improve the content
and distribution of information available to parents on
immunisation in its various forms since misunderstand-
ings and misinformation, in particular about immunisation for whooping cough and measles, still appear to be
widespread (Begg and White 1987; Morgan *et al* 1987).

In a move intended to encourage increased uptake of
immunisation, the new 1990 contract of service for
general practitioners (Health Departments of Great
Britain 1989) includes targets for childhood immunisation with payments for two levels of achievement across
three groups of immunisation—diphtheria, tetanus, and
poliomyelitis, pertussis, and mumps, measles, and

rubella. The higher level of payment will be made to GPs who achieve 90 per cent coverage and the lower payment to those who achieve at least 70 per cent cover. The same target levels will apply to pre-school boosters for children under 5 years of age. One practical problem with this is that of the denominator to be used in calculating rates of coverage since existing population registers are known to be inaccurate by about 20 per cent. There is a case to be made for transferring responsibility for all immunisations to general practitioners so that one clearly identified group of professionals would be responsible for encouraging uptake (Waller and Morgan 1988).

Macfarlane and Pillay (1984) confirmed the massive variation in the level of provision of child health surveillance and who provides it. In a national study they found that all child health clinics in Croydon were carried out by clinical medical officers, in East Suffolk 92 per cent of clinics were run by health visitors, and in Oxford, 73 per cent were run by general practitioners. They suggested that all involved should meet and agree a national policy of child health surveillance based on what was available and relevant, and that the policy should be continually evaluated.

VARIATION IN PROVISION AND CONTENT OF SERVICE

The involvement of so many different health personnel in this area is also a factor in the variation in provision of service between different parts of the country. Although, as we have said, there has been a long established tradition of child health surveillance, there has been no clearly stated and agreed national policy (Waller and Morgan 1988). The system has evolved in a patchy and unco-ordinated way rather than having been developed systematically. Macfarlane and Pillay (1984), for example, showed a six to seven-fold difference in the number of child health clinics per head of pre-school children (defined as those under 5 years of age) between Districts which did not seem to be related to demographic and social factors.

Nicoll (1984) found evidence, in deprived areas at least, of a decline in attendance at child health clinics after the age of a year and a half. Morgan and colleagues (1989), in an examination of the role of child health clinics in an inner London district, found that clinic attendance was frequent among all social groups in children aged under 6 months but declined thereafter. These workers found a sharp decline in clinic attendances once a child reached one year of age. They suggest that the main reason fo this is that by this time mothers are more confident of their own ability to cope and are no longer in need of such frequent support and reassurance.

There are wide variations also in the number of pre-school checks in both training and non-training general practices (Burke and Bain 1986). In some none were carried out, in some there were nine, and the mean number of checks was three. The Royal College of General Practitioners (1982) recommended four pre-school examinations carried out in special sessions in general practices with a health visitor also present. The College also recommended a routine check at the age of 12–13 years but only an estimated 2 per cent of practices were found to carry this out (Burke and Bain 1986). In the new contract of service for general practice (Health Departments of Great Britain 1989), suitably trained GPs will be able to offer child health surveillance services to any child under 5 years on their list at the following stages relevant to childhood as defined in this chapter—21 months (within the range 18–24 months) and 39 months (within the range 36–42 months).

There is also variation in the content of screening examinations in children. In 1983, the Royal College of General Practitioners listed the following items for inclusion in pre-school screening—congenital dislocation of the hip (CDH), maldescent of testes, squint, vision, hearing—since tests in these areas had been validated as effective and safe, and capable of being carried out in the primary care setting. They also described the kind of developmental examinations that should be carried out in relation to motor and language development. However, many of these tests have not been properly validated and, as mentioned in Chapter 2, routine screening for CDH remains controversial.

In a report of a study in Northumberland, Colver and Steiner (1986) emphasise the lack of a nationally agreed content for child surveillance and describe how discussions with every general practice, health visitor, and clinical medical officer in the Northumberland Health Authority led to agreement on the content of pre-school health surveillance, the age at which it should be done, and referral pathways after a positive screening test. Agreement was reached that child health clinics should include developmental guidance and health education, screening and assessment of any problems presented by parents or health visitors. It was felt that a battery of developmental screening tests were unhelpful because the range of normal is so wide, decisions depend too heavily on the clinical judgment of the observer, and a high level of anxiety can be generated in parents.

Non-attendance at clinics is a perennial problem and there is concern that those children in greatest need of surveillance and screening are least likely to undergo it (Waller and Morgan 1988). Houston and Davis (1985) found that children at highest risk tended to have more contact with their general practitioners than others and concluded that surveillance would be more effectively centred on these contacts than on expecting them to be brought to separate clinics for assessment although this would need some form of structured medical records to be completed opportunistically. It must be questioned also whether it applies to children in families who move frequently, such as travelling people, single parent families, and the socially deprived.

LACK OF SCIENTIFIC EVALUATION OF SCREENING PROGRAMMES

Evaluation, as we have stressed earlier and as cannot be over-emphasised, is an absolutely vital element in screening. A screening test may itself be effective while the screening service which uses it may not. Wald (1984) cites the example of screening for cervical cancer which has been shown to be an effective method of reducing the incidence of invasive cervical cancer. In Britain, however, the cervical cancer screening programme has failed in its objective so far. There is a vast difference between a programme of screening carried out in strict research conditions in a centre of excellence and a programme universally applied in routine practice. This distinction between whether screening for a particular disorder is worthwhile and whether screening programmes for that disorder work in practice is an important one.

This is very relevant in the difficult and often controversial context of child health surveillance and screening. Since there is a long established tradition of such activities and very little evaluation, certain examinations may be carried out routinely and rigorously with little benefit just because they have always been done, while other very basic screening procedures, such as listening to parental concerns, may be almost entirely neglected.

Thus, at this crucial early stage of life, there is in Britain at present no nationally agreed policy on surveillance and screening, considerable confusion over definitions, uncertainty over who does what, regional variation in provision, content, and standard of coverage, and at the least inadequate evaluation of what is being done.

WHAT CHILD HEALTH SCREENING IS WORTHWHILE?

In 1967 the Sheldon Report recommended the following functions of the child health service—routine medical examinations of children presumed to be healthy; infant nutrition and hygiene; detection of defects such as physical disorders, mental retardation, and emotional health; parental counselling; health education; measurements; immunisation and vaccination. It is thus over 30 years since this area of health work has been officially examined and the publication of the Hall report in 1989 provides a timely review of the subject (Polnay 1989). The Hall Working Party considered current screening procedures in children in detail and produced a recommended core programme of surveillance for all children to be undertaken by the primary health care team and incorporating those screening procedures which they believe can be supported in the light of the available evidence. A summary of their recommendations for the 1–11 year age group is given in Table 10. The recommendations concentrate heavily on basic surveillance of sight, hearing, and general behaviour and on parental and later teacher concerns and perceptions. This is a sound and practical approach, using the knowledge of those who know a particular child best. It is likely to work most effectively, however, with the more intelligent, perceptive, and committed parents whose children will be least at risk from failure to detect problems. Doubts have been expressed as to whether it will work as well in deprived inner city areas and in lower social class groups where need may be greatest (Bax and Whitmore 1990). However, as we discuss in relation to screening in adult women, there is some indication that screening may have more appeal when it is placed in the context of total health care rather than when the emphasis is placed on screening for particular diseases.

The Report considers seven groups of screening tests currently undertaken and we will deal briefly with the recommendations in each group together with results from other studies as appropriate.

TABLE 10. *Recommended regular screening procedures in childhood**

AGE (RANGE)	PROCEDURES
21 months (18–24 mo)	Enquire about parental concerns, particularly on behaviour, vision, and hearing. Do not attempt formal tests of vision or hearing—arrange detailed assessment if either are in doubt. Confirm child is walking with normal gait, is beginning to say words, and understands when spoken to. Remember high prevalence of iron deficiency anaemia at this age. Enquire about immunisation status.
39 months (36–42 mo)	Ask about vision, squint, hearing, behaviour, and development. Discuss with parent/s any concerns as to whether child may have any special educational problems or needs and arrange further action as appropriate. Measure height and plot on chart. Check for testicular descent in boys (if not checked on any other occasion since 8 mo). If indicated, perform or arrange hearing test. Enquire about immunisation status.
5 years (48–66 mo)	School entry. Ask about any parental or teacher concerns. Review pre-school records. Undertake physical examination, including auscultation of the heart, if specific indication or if no record is available to confirm previous medical care. Measure height and plot on chart. Check vision using Snellen chart. Check hearing by 'sweep' test. Enquire about immunisation status.
School years	Further tests of visual acuity at ages 8 and 11 years. Test colour vision using Ishihara plates at age 11 years. Repeat height measurement if indicated. Enquire about immunisation status.

*Adapted from *Health for All Children* (Hall 1989) and reproduced by kind permission of the authors and Oxford University Press.

1. The physical examination

According to the Hall recommendations, existing screening programmes, such as those for congenital dislocation of the hip and undescended testes, should continue, provided that data are being collected that will be useful in further evaluation. However successful programmes depend on satisfactory clinical skills and good organisation. New screening programmes should not be introduced at the present time. As we discussed in Chapter 2, however, the evidence of screening for congenital dislocation of the hip—at least in the neonatal period—is far from unequivocal.

2. Laboratory and Radiological Screening Tests

The only recommendation relevant to children in the age range under consideration in this chapter concerns iron deficiency anaemia. This is a common disorder with an apparent peak at around 3 years and an average prevalence of 5–10 per cent. The Report states that screening for iron deficiency anaemia is certainly possible and probably desirable but that published evidence to date allows of only one firm recommendation—that

> all staff need to be aware that iron deficiency is a very common disorder and one that is easily treated. There should be no hesitation about obtaining an Hb estimation and where necessary giving a therapeutic trial of iron.

Further research is needed and among questions to be considered are whether parents would find routine blood sampling for this purpose acceptable, whether the incidence of iron deficiency could be reduced by appropriate health education, and what measurable benefits might result from a more aggressive approach to the identification and treatment of iron deficiency?

James and colleagues (1988) describe a study of iron deficiency in their Bristol practice in an area of widespread social deprivation in which 537 children aged between 1 and 4 years were identified and parents informed of the importance of identifying and treating iron deficiency and invited to attend an iron clinic. Over the six months of the study, 365 of the eligible children were scanned (69·3 per cent.) Of these 58 (15·9 per cent) were iron deficient and 21 (5·8 per cent) anaemic. Caucasian children had a significantly lower incidence of iron deficiency than non-Caucasians. Afro-Caribbeans were the largest ethnic minority group and 24 per cent were iron deficient. This practice has now adopted a policy of screening all children for iron deficiency at 14 months when they attend for measles immunisation. On the basis of their experience, these general practitioners would encourage routine screening of all children.

Elwood (1988) on the other hand, feels that available evidence on the prevalence and importance of the condition indicates that screening for iron deficiency cannot be justified. He suggests that the identification and treatment of affected individuals should be part of normal clinical practice and emphasises the point that a low concentration of circulating haemoglobin can be a consequence of serious underlying disease. He acknowledges that infants and young children do merit special consideration because iron deficiency may be of importance in relation to normal growth and development. Case detection of anaemia in normal clinical practice should also be very efficient in this group because of the frequency with which they are seen by doctors and other health professionals. If any general measure directed to children is proposed, prevalence studies and randomised controlled trials of the effects of the measures proposed should be carried out first. However, doubts have been expressed by paediatricians themselves as to the advantage of such measures. Addy (1986) for example, suggests that the size of the problem needs to be properly assessed and that the best current approach might be to test infants at 9–12 months especially in socially underprivileged areas.

The US Preventive Services Task Force (1989) recommends screening all infants for anaemia once before they reach the age of 18 months. The Canadian Task Force (1979), however, does not support routine anaemia screening in children.

Once again there is no general agreement on screening for iron deficiency anaemia and important questions remain to be answered about the acceptability and effectiveness of intervention and screening (Polnay 1989).

3. Growth Monitoring

The US Preventive Services Task Force (1989) recommended that the height and weight of children should be measured regularly and plotted on a growth chart throughout infancy and childhood. They drew attention to the association between obesity and major chronic diseases such as diabetes and coronary heart disease and pointed out that such periodic measurements are inexpensive, rapid, and acceptable to patients. The Canadian Task Force (1979) recommended measurement of height, weight, and head circumference at ages 18 months, 2–3 years, 4 years, 5–6 years, and 10–11 years and thereafter at the clinician's discretion.

Weight. This is a firmly established routine procedure in babies in the United Kingdom but the Hall Working Party saw no reason for continuing it routinely beyond the first year of life. It is, however, a useful point of contact and discussion with parents who may then raise other worries and factors that might not otherwise be mentioned, and they recommended that children should be weighed on request.

Height. The screening test is the measurement itself which must be plotted on a chart. A height measurement should be made and recorded at around 3 years of age and again between 4 and 5 years. Beyond the age of 5 years, height should be measured only if there is doubt about the significance of previous measurements or if previous results are absent or unsatisfactory.

On the question of height, Price and colleagues (1988) reported a study of the height of primary schoolchildren and their parents' perceptions of food intolerance undertaken within a larger national study of health and growth. Children were categorised according to their experience of food intolerance on the basis of their parents' responses to a self-completed questionnaire. The heights of the children in each group were then compared. Useful responses to the questions of food intolerance were received from 6813 children in the sample (85 per cent) and measurements of height were obtained for 7856 (98 per cent). Children with food intolerance were shorter than other children—a difference in height of about 1·5 cm remained after adjusting for social and biological factors and some common symptoms in childhood. These workers suggest that, regardless of the underlying aetiology, parents' complaints of food intolerance in their children should be taken seriously

This is of interest here in that two simple screening devices of a self-completed questionnaire and a measurement of height can also be used to identify a possible area of concern. Other things being equal, growth, in terms of height, is a general measure of health. Food intolerance is still rather an imprecise term. Research is needed to determine prevalence and gain insight into processes but it seems clear that, in some children, there is a relationship between certain types of food and behavioural and developmental problems which is worth exploring. This study also emphasises the points brought out clearly in the Hall Report of the importance of involving, informing, and trusting the judgment of parents. There is no evidence to suggest that routine measurement of height and weight in perfectly normal children is worthwhile.

4. Screening for Sensory Impairments

Chamberlain (1984) includes sensory impairments in the small group of conditions for which screening is justified in this age group since simple corrective measures are of benefit with defects of both sight and hearing.

Sight. The Hall Report recommends that screening for visual defects in pre-school children should be confined to history and observation. Children with suspected defects, a significant family history or a neurological condition should be examined by a specialist. An inspection of the eyes to detect squint should be part of any paediatric examination. A test of visual acuity should be carried out at school entry and thereafter every three years. A screening test for colour vision should be performed between the ages of 9 and 13. While defective colour vision is not generally a serious problem, it may be important in consideration of appropriate career choices. One person in every health board or district should take responsibility for co-ordinating this service. We would agree with this recommendation.

The US Preventive Services Task Force (1989) re-commends vision screening for all children once before they enter school, preferably at the age of 3 or 4 years. Routine visual testing is not recommended by them as part of the periodic health examination of asymptomatic schoolchildren.

Ingram and colleagues (1986), in a report on a study of screening $3\frac{1}{2}$ year-old children for visual defects, found no evidence to support the suggestion that a national programme of vision screening at this age should be contemplated. Further critical assessment would be essential before any such decision was made.

The Court Report (1976) included the recommenda-tion that children should have their vision screened at $3\frac{1}{2}$ years on the grounds that squint and amblyopia would then be identified at an age when remedial treatment might be successful. However, although there have been a number of trials of screening children at this age, screening has never been continued for long enough to permit proper evaluation. And as Sackett and Holland (1975) have pointed out

> implementation of untested community screening or treatment renders their subsequent evaluation more difficult and less decisive... indeed it may become im-possible to correct the original error.

In a study of referral patterns after school entry

medical examinations, Rona and colleagues (1989) suggest that the comparatively large percentage of children not identified as having a visual impairment earlier can be attributed to the low sensitivity of the particular tests used at age $3\frac{1}{2}$ years and report a commitment in the health district involved to change the assessment test used.

Stewart-Brown and Haslum (1988) report the results of a survey of health district screening programmes for vision in school which took place at the end of 1984. The response rate from districts in England and Wales was 81 per cent. All 165 districts that responded screened for loss of distant visual acuity, 96 per cent screened for loss of colour vision, 73 per cent for squint, and 67 per cent for loss of near visual acuity. The frequency of screening varied considerably as did criteria for referral, and there was a lack of evaluation and monitoring. The results suggested that a high proportion of districts devote more resources to screening vision in schools than can be justified on the basis of likely benefit. There seem to be considerable scope for improving the effectiveness of these programmes by increasing reliability while reducing the frequency of screening.

Hearing. No universal screening test of hearing is recommended by the Hall Working Party between the first birthday and school entry. Whenever a pre-school child is seen, parents should be asked whether they have any concerns on hearing. Parental concern is a sufficient indication for diagnostic testing. The school entry sweep test of hearing should be continued although its limitations are recognised. No further routine test of hearing is recommended. Once again we would agree with this recommendation.

Screening is of no value unless comprehensive and reliable audiological diagnostic and treatment facilities are available, and, while this may sound like overstating the obvious, this is by no means the case over the United Kingdom as a whole.

This was also found to be an area of high variability between districts and health boards in terms of numbers of tests performed, referral policy, and access to treatment. There was also very little in the way of monitoring and evaluation. One person in every health board or district should take responsibility for co-ordinating the surveillance of hearing in childhood.

The US Preventive Services Task Force (1989) recommends that high-risk children not tested at birth should be screened for hearing impairment before the age of 3 years. Risk factors include family history of childhood hearing impairment, congenital perinatal infection with herpes, syphilis, rubella, cytomegalo-virus, or toxoplasmosis, malformations involving the head or neck, low birthweight, bacterial meningitis, hyperbilirubinaemia requiring exchange transfusion, or severe perinatal asphyxia. The Task Force suggests that there is insufficient evidence to recommend routine audiological testing of all children in this age group or beyond.

5. Developmental Screening

Developmental testing, including language and motor assessment, has traditionally formed a very important part of screening in childhood. It is unfortunately also one in which the level of evaluation has been minimal —it was 'thought' to be valuable and is often continued simply because 'it has always been done.' As Illing-worth (1989) has pointed out, one important reason for the limitation of developmental assessment is that only one small part of the child has been tested—his or her response to certain readily scorable items—when we need to study the child as a whole.

Rona, Allsop and Morris (1987) have drawn attention to some of the difficulties involved in administering and monitoring the developmental examination schedule in an inner city health district. They note that for the routine pre-school entry examination which takes place in most health districts and boards in the United Kingdom, there is no prescribed examination routine but 70 per cent include a developmental examination (Haines *et al* 1985).

The Hall Working Party found no justification for repeated routine developmental examination of all pre-school children and recommended that these be discontinued. They advocate a new approach relying more heavily on the role of parents in detecting and accepting developmental problems. The advantage of this approach is that, by eliminating developmental examinations in children where they are clearly unnecessary, more professional time can be released for those who really require expert help and support.

As already discussed in Chapter 2, this is one of the aspects of the Hall Report which has caused the most controversy. Wilson (1990) agrees that much routine repeated developmental testing is probably unnecessary as most experienced doctors will identify abnormal development by listening to parental concerns, taking family histories, and observing the children themselves. However, he cautions that less experienced practitioners will still learn best by using developmental check lists.

The point must also be reiterated that reliance on parental concerns about a child's development presupposes that that concern exists and can be articulated, and will inevitably leave a vulnerable minority of children uncovered. We would suggest, therefore, that any changes in the developmental testing of children should be evaluated first in one or two health authority areas to see whether the resources released could actually be successfully targetted to that vulnerable minority.

6. Screening for Psychiatric Disorders

Social and psychiatric problems are very common in childhood (Richman, Stevenson and Graham 1977, Earls 1980, Graham 1986). These include pre-school adjustment disorders, neurotic and behavioural disorders, eating disorders and so on. Pre-school adjustment disorders are of particular importance but although individual case studies suggest that treatment may be effective, there are no large-scale population studies to demonstrate the feasibility of providing intervention programmes in whole communities.

The Hall Working Party suggested that screening, using a check-list or questionnaire, can help to highlight problems and enable parents to recognise the existence of a behavioural difficulty. They recommended that these should not be used routinely but can be introduced in training programmes and in selected cases. Once again decisions about referral depend on discussion with parents, their willingness to use psychiatric or psychological help which unfortunately still carry something of a stigma, and the availability of adequate support and referral services which are very variable. There have been recent suggestions that psychiatrists might attend for sessions in group practices and this certainly seems an idea worth pursuing (Horder 1990).

SCREENING AND HEALTH EDUCATION

It can be argued that, at its most basic, screening can be nothing more than a simple question in appropriate circumstances. Wald (1984) for example, has suggested that the most basic screening test for Down syndrome is to ascertain maternal age.

One important area of child health care where screening at this basic level would be relevant is that of immunisation (Senturia and Peckham 1987, Jarman et al 1988). Infections and parasitic diseases still account for over 7 per cent of all deaths in the 1–4 year age group in England and Wales and, as we have already mentioned, even where the results of these illnesses are not so dramatic, sequelae and foundations of future ill health are also relevant. A more positive approach to immunisation would require more factual information available to both parents and health professionals but the benefits of increasing uptake should surely merit the inclusion of a basic screening question on immunisation status in any health contact concerning a child of the appropriate age. In this respect the new GP contract may be helpful in encouraging a more positive approach on the part of general practitioners.

SUMMARY AND CONCLUSIONS

The current state of screening in what we define here as childhood is characterised by confusion and diversity (Butler 1989). There is a woeful lack of research and evaluation, very variable provision, content, and quality of screening services, and little overall co-ordination. Yet the benefits of screening are more evident early in life and the target group is easily defined and mostly in regular contact with the health system.

The Working Group on Health Surveillance in Children (Hall 1989) has in our view provided a welcome and overdue review which looks at what is happening, reports it coherently and comprehensively, and makes clear recommendations. The Report has three main thrusts as summarised by Polnay (1989). Firstly, it argues that the content of the screening programme should be determined by our state of knowledge about the conditions sought, the effectiveness of the test, and the availability of programmes for management. Secondly, it emphasises that parents are far more effective than professionals in the early diagnosis of a wide range of handicaps. Thirdly, it underlines and clarifies the health education content of the surveillance programme. As we have already described, there have been criticisms—most notably about the definitions and confusion between screening and surveillance and about the children at risk who may remain outside the health care network. We would also caution that even the most caring and alert of parents may not identify a potentially serious development or health problem, such as for example, a heart murmur, before it begins to cause problems or symptoms.

It must also be remembered that, in the past, many of the most dramatic improvements in public health came as a result of better social and economic conditions and such simple environmental activities as improving the water supply and cleaning up the air, rather than as a response to direct medical action. As Bain (1989) points out

> In the midst of pleas for more and more medical intervention, it is worth remembering that the main factors which have a significant effect on childhood morbidity and mortality are poverty and accidents.

In practice, we believe that the Hall Report provides guidelines for the development of an excellent system of surveillance and screening in childhood as summarised in Table 10. As Colver (1990) has suggested, there would be much to be gained from implementing the report's recommendations across the country,

> the alternative is for each district or primary health care team to continue to adhere to its own judgements and prejudices in the vain hope that it has found the perfect programme and can implement and evaluate it.

It is surely time to adopt a more practical and systematic approach to screening in this age group. More evaluation and better co-ordination are essential to the achievement of national standards with emphasis on the role of screening in prevention with effective health education and encouragement towards increased uptake of immunisation. Only in this way can screening and surveillance in children become what they already are in the best of general practices—part of normal health care that can be expected by every family.

REFERENCES

ADDY, D. P. 'Happiness is: iron'. *Br Med J* 1986, 292:969–70.

BAIN, J. 'Developmental screening for pre-school children: is it worthwhile? *J Roy Coll Gen Practit* 1989, 39:133–7.

BARKER, D. J. P. AND OSMOND, C. 'Childhood respiratory infection and adult chronic bronchitis in England and Wales'. *Br Med J* 1986, 293:1271–5.

BAX, M. C. O. AND WHITMORE, K. 'Health for all children'. (Book review). *Arch Dis Child* 1990, 65:141–2.

BEGG, N. T. AND NOAH, N. D. 'Immunisation targets in Europe and Britain'. *Br Med J* 1985, 291:1370–1.

BEGG, N. AND WHITE, J. *A survey of pre-school immunisation programmes in England and Wales.* London: Public Health Laboratory Service, 1987.

BURKE, P. AND BAIN, J. 'Paediatric developmental screening: a survey of general practitioners'. *J Roy Coll Gen Practit* 1986, 36:302–6.

BUTLER, J. R. *Child Health Surveillance in Primary Care: A Critical Review.* London: HMSO, 1989.

CANADIAN TASK FORCE. 'The periodic health examination'. *Can Med Assoc J* 1979, 121:1194–1254.

CHAMBERLAIN, JOCELYN, M. 'Which prescriptive screening programmes are worthwhile? *J Epidemiol Comm Hlth* 1984, 38:270–7.

COLVER, A. 'Health for all children'. (Book review). *Arch Dis Child* 1990, 65:142.

COLVER, A. F. AND STEINER, H. 'Health surveillance of pre-school children'. *Br Med J* 1986, 293:258–60.

THE COURT REPORT. Committee on Child Health Services. *Fit for the Future.* Cmnd 6684. London: HMSO, 1968.

DHSS. *Vaccination and immunization rates for England 1985.* London: DHSS, 1986.

EARLS, F. 'Prevalence of behaviour problems in three-year-old children. A cross-national replication'. *Arch Gen Psychiatr* 1980, 37:1153–7.

ELWOOD, P. C. 'Iron deficiency'. In *Elimination or Reduction of Diseases.* ALAN J. SILMAN AND SHANE P. A. ALLWRIGHT (eds) pp. 126–39. Oxford: Oxford University Press, 1988.

GRAHAM, P. 'Pre-school behavioural adjustment disorders'. In: *Child Psychiatry. A Developmental Approach.* P. J. GRAHAM (ed.) pp. 80–3. Oxford: Oxford University Press 1986.

HAINES, C. R., BROWN, J. B., GRANTHAM, E. B., RAJAGOPOLAN, V. S., AND SUTCLIFFE, P. V. 'Neurodevelopmental screening in the school entrant medical examination as a predictor of co-ordination and communication difficulties'. *Arch Dis Child* 1985, 60:1122–7.

HALL, DAVID, M. B. (ed.) *Health for All Children: A programme of Child Health Surveillance.* Report of the Joint Working Party on Child Health Surveillance. Oxford: Oxford University Press, 1989.

HEALTH DEPARTMENTS OF GREAT BRITAIN. *General Practice in the National Health Service. The 1990 Contract.* London: Health Departments of Great Britain, 1989.

HOLLAND, W. W. AND REID, D. D. 'The urban factor in chronic bronchitis'. *Lancet* 1965, i:445–44.

HORDER, J. Personal communication, 1990.

HOUSTON, H. L. A. AND DAVIS, R. H. 'Opportunistic surveillance of child development in primary care: is it feasible?' *J Roy Coll Gen Practit* 1985, 35:77–9.

ILLINGWORTH, R. S.'Trying to understand development'. In *Early Influences Shaping the Individual*. S. DOXIADIS (ed.) New York and London: Plenum Press, 1989.

INGRAM, R. M., HOLLAND, W. W., WALKER, C., WILSON, J. M. ARNOLD, P. E. AND DALY, S. 'Screening for visual defects in pre-school children'. *Br J Ophthalmol* 1986, 70:16–21.

JAMES, J., EVANS, J., MALE, P., PALLISTER, C., HENDRIKZ, J. K. AND OAKHILL, A. Iron deficiency in inner city pre-school children: development of a general practice screening programme'. *J Roy Coll Gen Practit* 1988, 38:250–2.

JARMAN, B., BOSANQUET, N., RICE, P., DOLLIMORE, N. AND LEESE, B. 'Uptake of immunization in district health authorities in England'. *Br Med J* 1988, 296:1775–8.

Lancet (editorial). 'Immunization policy: recipes for success'. *Lancet* 1987, 2:78–80.

MACFARLANE, J. A. AND PILLAY, U. 'Who does what and how much in the pre-school child health services in England?' *Br Med J* 1984, 289:851–2.

MORGAN, M., LAKHANI, A. D., MORRIS, R. W., DALE, C. AND VAILE, M. S. B. 'Parents' attitudes to measles immunisation'. *J Roy Coll Gen Practit* 1987, 37:25–7.

MORGAN, M., REYNOLDS, A., MORRIS, R., ALLSOP, M. AND RONA, R. 'Who uses child health clinics and why: a study of a deprived inner city district'. *Health Visitor* 1989: 62:244–7.

NICOLL, A. 'The value of selective pre-school medicals in an inner-city area'. *Publ Hlth Lond* 1984, 98:68–72.

POLNAY, L. 'Child health surveillance'. *Br Med J* 1989, 289:1351–2.

PRICE, C. E., RONA, R. J. AND CHINN, S. 'Height of primary schoolchildren and parents' perception of food intolerance'. *Br Med J* 1988, 296:1696–9.

RICHMAN, N., STEVENSON, J. AND GRAHAM P. 'Prevalence of behaviour problems in pre-school children: an epidemiological study in a London borough'. *J Child Psychol Psychiatr* 1977, 16:277–87.

RONA, R. J., ALLSOP, M. AND MORRIS, R. W. 'Monitoring the developmental examination schedule in an inner city health district'. *Childcare, Health and Development*, 1987, 13:329–40.

RONA, R. J. ALLSOP, M., MORRIS, R. AND MORGAN, M. 'Referral patterns after school medical examinations'. *Arch Dis Child* 1989, 64:829–33.

ROYAL COLLEGE OF GENERAL PRACTITIONERS. *Healthier Children—thinking Prevention*. London, 1982.

ROYAL COLLEGE OF GENERAL PRACTITIONERS. *Promoting Prevention*. Occasional paper No. 22. London, 1983.

SACKETT, D. L. AND HOLLAND, W. W. 'Controversy in the detection of disease'. *Lancet* 1975, 2:357–9.

SENTURIA, Y. D. AND PECKHAM, C. S. 'Pre-school immunization: the importance of achieving adequate uptake'. *Children and Society* 1987, 1:198–209.

STEWART-BROWN, S. L. AND HASLUM, M. 'Screening of vision in school: could we do better by doing less?' *Br Med J* 1988, 297:1111–13.

US PREVENTIVE SERVICES TASK FORCE. *Guide to Clinical Preventive Services. An Assessment of the Effectiveness of 169 Interventions.* Baltimore: Williams and Wilkins, 1989.

WALD, N. J. (ed.) *Antenatal and Neonatal Screening.* Oxford: Oxford University Press, 1984.

WALLER, JANE AND MORGAN, MYFANWY. *The Use of Preventive Measures in Primary Care. Report prepared for the World Health Organization.* 1988.

WILSON, J. A. 'Health for all children'. (Book review). *Arch Dis Child* 1990, 65:142.

4 SCREENING IN ADOLESCENCE AND EARLY ADULTHOOD

I would there were no age between ten and
three and twenty, or that youth would sleep
out the rest; for there is nothing in the
between but getting wenches with child,
wronging the ancientry, stealing, fighting
(SHAKESPEARE: *The Winter's Tale*)

INTRODUCTION

THE YEARS FROM 12 TO 24 WHICH COVER OUR LIFE CYCLE
periods of adolescence and early adulthood are ones in
which formal contact with the health service is for most
people at its lowest level during a lifetime. But problems
exist. This period has been described as a process of
movement from a condition of relative dependence on
adults to one of autonomy (Spicer 1990). It is without
question a very difficult time of life. Adolescents are
coping with profound physical and emotional changes
which are bound to affect them to a greater or lesser
degree. They want freedom but often lack the experience and judgment to use it widely.

> The contrariness of adolescents is notorious: they are
> hypochondriacal yet mistrust doctors; they need support
> and collaboration from parents and teachers but go out of
> their way to make this difficult.

Spicer (1990) has discussed some of the difficulties
and problem areas relevant to this age group and these
are summarised in Table 11. Health education and
preventive medicine should be of particular importance
during adolescence since this is a time of life when good
health habits can be established but when personal
stresses and external and peer group pressure can
persuade otherwise—as, for example, with alcohol,
drug, or solvent abuse. Because of the special charac-

98

TABLE 11. *Nine problem areas in adolescence and early adulthood**

1 Excessive consumption of alcohol, use of drugs, solvent abuse
2 Delinquency and aggressive behaviour
3 Running away from home and drifting
4 Promiscuous sexual behaviour, pregnancy, and venereal disease
5 Depression or anxiety and inability to work or study
6 Withdrawal from relationships and loneliness
7 Risk to life by fast driving of motor vehicles
8 Anorexia and other disorders of feeding
9 Drug overdose and attempted suicide

*From Spicer (1990) and reproduced by kind permission of the author and Oxford University Press.

teristics of adolescents, however, many may be reluctant to seek advice and help through conventional health channels. At this age, it may be easier to trust and discuss personal and sensitive matters, such as aspects of sexual and emotional development or troubled family relationships, with someone outside the existing medical or family framework. General practitioners, however, are well placed to offer advice and support during routine consultation. Understanding and respected teachers can also provide a great deal of support in this context although some adolescents need to discuss problems with someone absolutely separate from the family. Youth counselling and advisory services now exist throughout Britain and Europe although provision and quality vary widely (WHO 1977). The media too can be a potent source of influence for good or ill. Some programmes or advertisements provide a negative model—for example, the glamorous image often portrayed of consuming alcohol or driving fast cars—or fuel unrealistic aspirations and expectations which cannot be fulfilled. On the positive side, the problem pages of youth magazines and the increasing number of help lines on local radio give troubled youngsters the chance to discuss problems without the need for formal consultation. Spicer (1990) mentions the

London radio station, Capital Radio, which has specific 'help lines' for young people, offering advice on practical, emotional, and sexual problems both over the phone and at base. Opportunities for advice and help on health and related matters in adolescence and early adulthood are shown in Table 12.

TABLE 12. *Opportunities for advice and help on health and related matters in adolescence and early adulthood*

LOCATION	TYPE OF HEALTH PROFESSIONAL
General practice	GP, health visitor, practice nurse
Hospital	Specialist medical or paramedical hospital staff as appropriate
School	Clinical medical officer, school nurse, dentist, educational psychologist, speech therapist, teacher
Further education	Student health centre and counselling service
Community	Clinical medical officer, dentist, optometrist, pharmacist, youth counselling services, newspaper and magazine problem pages, local radio help lines, family planning clinic
Employment	Occupational medical officer, works nurse

We do not consider that it would be beneficial to advocate formal screening for any specific conditions during this period when compliance would be likely to present even more of a problem than it does in other age groups. We would advocate instead the strengthening of informal advice centres for young people where they could discuss matters with skilled people perceived as non-authoritarian and non-judgmental. In this chapter we will discuss the current evidence on screening for scoliosis, one of the few conditions currently the subject of screening in adolescence, immunity to rubella where a case could be made for screening adolescent girls until the disease ceases to be a threat, health education and promotion with particular reference to road accidents and suicide, sex education and family planning, and health-damaging behaviour, and finally screening for human immunodeficiency virus.

SCOLIOSIS

Screening for scoliosis in adolescents is one area of considerable current debate. The procedure suggested in the United Kingdom is visual inspection followed where necessary by X-ray (Chamberlain 1984). About 2 per cent of children are found to have some degree of scoliosis but only 0·2 per cent to require treatment by spinal brace or fusion. There is considerable doubt about the efficacy of treatment and evaluation is clearly vital.

A prevalence study of idiopathic scoliosis among 29,195 school children in Quebec was designed to determine whether a permanent screening programme for the condition was justified (Morais, Bernier and Turcotte 1985). The prevalence of the condition was 42·0 per 1000 in the screened population, 51·9 per 1000 in girls and 32·0 per 1000 in boys. Morais and her colleagues concluded that mass screening for idiopathic scoliosis does not seem to be justified in the present state of knowledge of the disease. They emphasise that the forward bending test produces not only large numbers of false positives, but a fair number of true positives who may never need treatment. These children may be unnecessarily exposed to X-rays and even treatment by brace or traction. The screening goal of early detection of asymptomatic health problems to provide effective treatment that will alter the prognosis favourably is not attainable with current screening techniques. Minor cases which are likely to progress need to be capable of distinction from those which will never become health problems.

Berwick (1985) draws attention to the fact that the vast majority of children with positive forward bending tests on scoliosis screening have curvatures of no current or future significance yet they are identified and labelled as having an abnormality. If scoliosis is defined as a curvature which will compromise function or appearance without treatment, almost all children with positive scoliosis screening results are false positives. In the Quebec study 51·7 per cent of the children with scoliosis were advised to do exercises. Yet the effectiveness of exercise in this condition has not been properly evaluated. Berwick concludes:

> To make rational policy, we at least need better data on the psychological morbidity for false positives, the effectiveness of treatment of moderate curves, the worth of exercises, and the marginal contribution of screening compared with spontaneous detection rates. Without such data, the hunt is as likely to be leading us into the swamp as towards our quarry.

An editorial in *The Lancet* (1988) draws attention to work on scoliosis screening by Guang-po and colleagues (1988) who followed a three-stage procedure in a prevalence study of screening in schools in China. The first stage was physical inspection and forward bending. The second stage was examination by Moire topography, a photographic technique to define body contours. Only those found to have a positive result by this test were referred for the third stage of radiography. These workers concluded that the use of Moire topography as a secondary screening procedure for scoliosis may reduce the number of cases referred for radiography.

The Hall Report (1989) confirms that the forward bending test is too sensitive and results in the unnecessary treatment of perhaps two out of every three children treated. Scoliosis is a condition which appears after the age of 10 years and is much more likely to progress to serious deformity in girls. The estimated incidence of scoliosis requiring treatment is around 3 per 1000. When progression does occur it affects lung and cardiac function and leads to severe cosmetic deformity (British Orthopaedic Association and British Scoliosis Society 1983). The Hall Working Group recommended that new screening programmes should not be introduced at present. All health care staff should be aware of the possible significance of scoliosis and the need for referral for orthopaedic opinion. Screening programmes currently in progress should continue provided that data are being collected for further evaluation.

In our view, this is an area which should be approached with extreme caution. If as is suggested, two out of every three children treated are being treated unnecessarily, this is simply not acceptable. Given the emotional minefield of adolescence, it is surely lunacy to risk labelling a child as having a condition unless the diagnosis is absolutely certain. Even if the only treatment available in less severe cases is exercise, this will present another avenue of potential conflict between a parent conscientiously trying to ensure that the exercise schedule is fulfilled and the sensitive and possibly rebellious adolescent. As mentioned above, it is by no means clear that exercise actually does any good. It also seems likely that almost all cases of scoliosis severe enough to require treatment will be identified by a parent, teacher, or in a routine health consultation in school or general practice.

RUBELLA

Rubella itself is a worldwide viral disease which is usually mild and in which complications are exceptional. It becomes important when contracted in early pregnancy when it can cause serious damage to the developing fetus. Individuals are protected from rubella by immunisation which in turn will reduce or eradicate congenital rubella syndrome. It has been estimated that, in the absence of control measures, the frequency of congenital rubella syndrome varies from 0·2 cases per 1000 births in a non-epidemic period to 2·0 cases per

1000 births during an epidemic (Knox 1980; Stray-Pedersen 1982).

In any discussion of immunisation for rubella it is vital to consider the strategy selected by the country concerned towards the disease. There are two main immunisation strategies for preventing rubella infection during pregnancy and these have been summarised by De Wals and Lechat (1988). The selective approach aims to protect susceptible women of child-bearing age without interfering with the transmission of the virus in the child population and the acquisition of natural immunity. This was the policy adopted in all European countries in the early 1970s. The mass or universal strategy aims to interrupt the spread of rubella by the immunisation of all children. Thus non-immunised women are protected from exposure itself rather than from the effects of exposure, and this was the approach adopted in the United States and Canada.

In the United Kingdom, current Department of Health guidelines on the use of the measles, mumps, and rubella vaccine (DHSS 1988) recommend immunisation of children of both sexes at age 1–2 years and children of both sexes at age 4–5 years before entry to primary school unless there is a record of a previous immunisation, a valid contra-indication, or laboratory evidence of immunity. In addition, rubella immunisation for girls aged 10–14 years should continue, with single antigen rubella vaccine and the present target of 95 per cent coverage. They also recommend the continuation of immunisation of non-immune women before pregnancy and after delivery. The immunisation acceptance rate among schoolgirls is currently 85 per cent (De Wals and Lechat).

In countries, such as the United States, which have adopted universal immunisation of both sexes as a strategy, high levels of uptake will eliminate the virus and with it the disease. Total success may depend on compulsion which seems to be more acceptable in the United States than it is likely to be in Europe. However, if eradication is not achieved, the risks to the non-immunised section of the population are substantial and, in some circumstances, a failed eradication programme will cause more cases of congenital rubella syndrome than it prevents. The benefits are high but so are the risks (Knox 1980, 1984, 1987).

A combination of the two strategies can be effective as long as a high level of immunisation of young children is achieved. In Sweden, for example, all 18 month old children are immunised with combined measles, mumps, and rubella vaccine and girls only are re-immunised at the age of 12 years (Christenson et al 1983).

A practical point related to compliance has been discussed by Thompson (1988). In a discussion of immunisation technique, he suggested that the general 90 per cent target is ambitious, given the 1986 uptake for measles immunisation in England and Wales of 71 per cent. He maintains that the site of immunisation has some bearing on uptake. The officially recommended site is the anterolateral aspect of the thigh or the upper arm. However, since 1974, he and his colleagues in three practices covering 20,000 patients have achieved 98 per cent uptake of immunisation administered into the buttocks of infants by state registered nurses. In 1985, there was disruption to the programme after an official complaint to the nurses that they were not using the formally recommended route. Thompson traced the basis for the official recommendation back to a paper published in 1961 which described evidence from dissection of a stillborn infant that a 38 mm needle inserted obliquely into the buttock could puncture the sciatic nerve (Gilles and French 1961). As Thompson points out, the needles used now are only 16 mm long and cannot reach the sciatic nerve. The belief therefore that using this site can damage the sciatic nerve is a 'myth from the era of plus fours and musical evenings,' and an infant placed across the mother's lap and held by her will not witness any assault and will be spared a great deal of unnecessary distress. Thompson states in conclusion

We have learnt from mothers in a working class practice
that it is pain, distress, and struggle that are the main
reasons for failing to return for reinforcement... I suggest
that the panic we commonly see, even in girls aged 10–14
attending for rubella vaccine, is due to a resurgence of
infantile fear experienced before intellectual resources to
control it were developed. In my opinion national hopes
need to rely on generally applying the best techniques.

This is an important practical point and raises the wider
issues, stressed elsewhere, of the need to examine the
basis for all procedures and not simply accept something as valid because it has 'always been done' in a
particular way.

A case could be made in the short term, until the
present immunisation strategies achieve an acceptably
high level of uptake and have been running long enough
to have an effect, for screening adolescent girls serolo-
gically for immunity to the rubella virus and immunising the non-immune. However, a more realistic approach in our view is to improve awareness of the
potential dangers of rubella and increase voluntary
acceptance of immunisation through using the best
techniques and better communication by health professionals, especially in high-risk groups such as ethnic
minorities and the socially disadvantaged. It should
perhaps be possible to test immunity at family planning
consultations and provide immunisation where necessary.

HEALTH EDUCATION AND PROMOTION

The age group 15–24 years, as adolescence merges into
early adulthood, is a time when physical and mental
faculties are at their peak. Individuals are beginning to
break away from their roots—physically in some cases
with a move to further education or employment
elsewhere—and emotionally in departing often from
the accepted values and standards of their parents to
develop their own lives and lifestyles. It is also a time of

maximum vulnerability and potential stress and this is reflected in the causes of death in this age group as shown in Table 13.

TABLE 13. *Main causes of death at ages 15–24 years (England and Wales 1986)*

CAUSE	NUMBER		% TOTAL DEATHS	
MALES				
External causes				
Motor vehicle accidents	1213		38·2	
Suicide	361	2159	11·4	68·0
Others	585		18·4	
Malignant disease	283		8·9	
Diseases of the nervous system				
including mental disorders	244		7·7	
Circulatory disease	173		5·4	
Respiratory disease	89		2·8	
Other causes	227		7.1	
	3175		99·9	
FEMALES				
External causes				
Motor vehicle accidents	291		23·6	
Suicide	78	566	6·3	45·8
Others	197		15·9	
Malignant disease	192		15·5	
Diseases of the nervous system				
including mental disorders	95		7·7	
Circulatory disease	71		5·7	
Respiratory disease	60		4.9	
Other causes	252		20·4	
	1236		100·0	

The main cause of death is from motor vehicle accidents, suicide, and other external causes, an appallingly high figure, particularly in males. As Spicer (1990) points out, almost half of all male deaths in this age group are caused by road accidents and the most important external factor is alcohol.

The figure for deaths from suicide is also an indication

that there is a need to consider carefully how best to provide help and relief from stress at this time of life. The American Academy of Pediatrics, for example, recommends asking all adolescents about suicidal thoughts during the routine medical history (American Academy of Pediatrics Committee on Adolescence 1988).

Sex education and family planning is another area which needs careful and sensitive handling with attention to more than the purely physiological aspects.

Some information is of course provided at school but again quality and depth is very variable.

Health-damaging habits, such as drug, alcohol, and solvent abuse, are also relevant in any consideration of health education at this time but once again this must be sensitively handled if it is not to encourage the very behaviour it is intended to prevent.

Spicer (1990) stresses the need for the further development of youth counselling and advisory services in addition to the more conventional sources of advice such as general practitioners or school staff. There has been a rapid expansion over the last 20 years in what are sometimes described as 'drop-in' centres for the young. Their aims, objectives, staffing, and funding are variable but they do provide an informality—in that young people can attend without referral and for a variety of reasons—and confidentiality that are particularly appealing to this age group. Television is another potent and ubiquitous source of information as is the personal example shown by well-known personalities, such as football players or pop stars with whom adolescents identify.

We would suggest that the general practitioner also has a very important role to play at this stage. Many adolescents and young adults do perceive their family doctor as a trusted source of advice and consult for various reasons including family planning, skin problems, acute respiratory illness and so on (Morrell 1990). All these consultations, handled sensitively, do provide opportunities for health education and screening.

HUMAN IMMUNODEFICIENCY VIRUS (HIV)

One area of screening which is obviously not confined to this age group but which first becomes generally relevant within it, is screening for human immunodeficiency virus (HIV), already discussed briefly in Chapter 2. This is another issue of much current controversy, and there is no national policy although HIV screening would serve one of the purposes originally proposed for screening— namely, protecting the public health (Wilson 1990). The detection of HIV infection in individuals presenting for advice is now straightforward. The enzyme-immunoassay HIV antibody tests have over 99 per cent sensitivity and specificity and, if used in combination, virtually guarantee a true result (Johnson and Griffiths 1989). Benefits for those found to be sero-positive include long-term follow-up and management, early diagnosis and treatment of opportunistic infections, counselling on safer sexual behaviour to reduce the risk of transmission, possibility of psychological adjustment before the onset of illness, the choice of participating in the current trials of zidovudine (AZT).

However, even when the specificity of a test is high, some who are truly without disease will be test positive (Weiss and Thier 1988).

> The potential consequences of incorrectly informing a person that he or she is infected with HIV are severe; certainly anguish, fear, and depression; perhaps lost jobs, denied applications for health insurance, or aborted pregnancies; possibly suicide.

Further, some infected individuals will also be seronegative at the time they are tested.

In 1987 Meyer and Pauker advised caution on the consequences of widespread screening for HIV. Screening blood donors prevents most transmission by this route because infected blood is not used. But how much does screening change behaviour? The evidence suggests that by no means all seropositive people practice safer sex and apparently only a minority abstain from childbearing (Wofsy 1987). Despite educational efforts, public understanding of AIDS remains limited. Screening individuals who have not asked to be tested for HIV infection remains highly controversial.

In 1987 Sir Richard Doll proposed anonymous screening for the prevalence of AIDS on blood samples taken in hospitals for other purposes. After samples had been tested for the reasons for which they were taken, all identification apart from donor's age, sex, and residential district would be removed and they would be tested for antibody to HIV. The epidemiological arguments for such prevalence studies are straightforward—HIV positivity occurs much earlier than AIDS and screening for prevalence of HIV would provide the earliest indication of spread within a population.

Despite initial rejection of the anonymous testing scheme (DHSS 1988), the British Government has now accepted the proposals to test anonymously blood samples obtained for other purposes. As mentioned in Chapter 2, from January 1990 excess blood taken from patients attending several genitourinary and antenatal clinics in England and Wales is being tested for the virus in a programme run by the Medical Research Council. Patients will not be asked for consent but participating clinics will clearly inform those attending of their policy and patients may opt out if they wish. Anyone who wants to know their HIV status may request testing in the normal way. As Gill, Adler, and Day (1989) point out, in a review of the scientific, legal, and ethical basis for the programme, this is an important step towards improving the understanding of the spread of HIV.

Gillon (1987), however, highlighted two ethical objections to anonymous testing—firstly, the testing would be carried out without the patient's permission and secondly, patients could not be informed of their HIV status even if they wanted to know. There is also the crucial point that screening for HIV does not fulfil one of the basic requirements of any screening technique—namely that there should be a proven and effective treatment available. Results of the current multi-centre trials of AZT may change this.

We would not advocate general screening for HIV in adolescence or any other period of life. In England the Health Education Authority includes HIV/Aids and Sexual Health as one of the programmes in its Strategic Plan for the next five years (HEA 1989), with young people as one of its priority target groups. Information on the risks of certain types of behaviour and the seriousness of the virus should be made available to adolescents and young adults at every opportunity and by all available means. General practitioners, are in a strong position to provide advice and screening for what may be described as the 'worried well'—for example, homosexuals who present with headache or a skin infection.

SUMMARY AND CONCLUSIONS

There are no formal screening programmes that we would consider to be relevant or necessary in this age group. Current screening programmes for scoliosis should be subject to scientific evaluation since there is evidence that many children are being treated unnecessarily. It also seems likely that cases of scoliosis of sufficient severity to need treatment will be identified at home, at school, or in normal health consultation. With immunity to rubella, uptake of MMR is now good in young children and efforts in adolescent and young adult girls should be devoted to improving awareness of the potential dangers of the virus in pregnancy and providing immunisation as necessary. In the absence of an effective treatment, screening for HIV cannot be recommended although we do support the anonymous testing currently underway which should make an important contribution to our understanding of the spread of the virus.

Screening at this stage of the life-cycle should be carried out opportunistically during routine consultation with the general practitioner or other member of the practice team which may also provide openings for health education and discussion on particular problems. Resources should also be devoted to providing appropriate and sufficient skilled counselling, support, and health education services in a way that is acceptable to young people to help them bridge the difficult gap between childhood and maturity. It is also important to remember that adolescents have rights as well as obligations and that any services for this age group should reflect this.

REFERENCES

AMERICAN ACADEMY OF PEDIATRICS COMMITTEE ON ADOLESCENCE. Suicide and suicide attempts in adolescents and young adults'. *Pediatrics* 1988, 81:322–4.

BERWICK, DONALD M. 'Scoliosis screening': a pause in the chase'. *Am J Publ Hlth* 1985, 75:1373–4.

THE BRITISH ORTHOPAEDIC ASSOCIATION AND THE BRITISH SCOLIOSIS SOCIETY. School screening for scoliosis'. *Br Med J* 1983, 287:963–4.

CHAMBERLAIN, JOCELYN M. 'Which prescriptive screening programmes are worthwhile?' *J Epideniol comm Hlth* 1984, 38:270–7.

CHRISTENSON, B., BOTTIGER, M. AND HELLER, L. Mass vaccination programme aimed at eradicating measles, mumps and rubella in Sweden: first experience'. *Br Med J* 1983, 287:389–91.

DE WALS, P AND LECHAT, M. 'Congenital rubella'. In *Elimination or Reduction of Diseases: Opportunities for Health Service Action in Europe.* A. J. SILMAN AND SHANE P. A. ALLWRIGHT, (eds) Oxford: Oxford University Press, Medical Publications, 1988.

DHSS. *Report of a Working group on the monitoring and surveillance of HIV infection and AIDS.* London: HMSO, 1988.

DHSS. *Immunisation against infectious disease.* London: DHSS, 1988.

DOLL, SIR RICHARD. 'A proposal for doing prevalence studies of AIDS'. *Br Med J* 1987, 294:244–24.

GILL, O. N., ADLER, M. W. AND DAY, N. E. 'Monitoring the prevalence of HIV. Foundations for a programme of unlinked anonymous testing in England and Wales'. *Br Med J* 1989, 299:1295–8.

GILLES, F. H. AND FRENCH, J. H. 'Postinjection sciatic nerve palsies in infants and children'. *J Pediatr* 1961, 38:195–204.

GILLON, R. 'Testing for HIV without permission'. *Br Med J* 1987, 294:821–3.

GUANG-PO, Z., ZI-RONG, L., XIN-RONG, W., WONG-LIAN, C. AND QUN-LI, C. 'Screening for scoliosis among schoolchildren in Beijing'. *Chinese Med J* 1988, 101:151–4.

HALL, DAVID M. B. (ed.) *Health for All Children: A programme of Child Health Surveillance. Report of the Joint Working Party on Child Health Surveillance.* Oxford: Oxford University Press, 1989.

HEALTH EDUCATION AUTHORITY. *Strategic Plan 1990–1995.* London: HEA, 1989.

JOHNSON, M. A. AND Griffiths, P. 'Screening for HIV'. *Br J Hosp Med* 1989, 41:119.

KNOX, E. G. 'Strategy for rubella vaccination'. *Int J Epidemiol* 1980, 9:13–23.

KNOX, E. G. 'Theoretical aspects of rubella vaccination strategies'. *Int J Infect Dis* 1984, 7:194–7.

KNOX, E. G. 'Personal and public health care: conflict, congruence or accommodation'. In *Ethical Dilemmas in Health Promotion.* S. DOXIADIS (ed.) Chichester: John Wiley and Sons, 1987.

Lancet editorial. 'School screening for scoliosis'. *Lancet* 1988, 2:378.

MEYER, K. B. AND PAUKER, S. G. 'Screening for HIV: can we afford the false positive rate?' *N Engl J Med* 1987, 318:238–41.

MORAIS, THERESE, BERNIER, MICHAELE, AND TURCOTTE, FERNAND. 'Age and sex-specific prevalence of scoliosis and the value of school screening programmes'. *Am J Publ Hlth* 1985, 75(12):1377–80.

MORRELL, D. *The Art of General Practice.* Fourth Edition. Oxford: Oxford University Press, 1991.

SPICER, R. F. 'Adolescents'. In *Oxford Textbook of Public Health,* 2nd edition. W. W. HOLLAND, R. DETELS AND E. G. KNOX (eds) Volume 3. Section D. Needs of Special Client Groups. Oxford: Oxford University Press, 1990.

STRAY-PEDERSEN, B. 'Economic evaluation of different vaccination programmes to prevent congenital rubella'. *NIPH Annals* 1982, 5:69–83.

THOMPSON, M. KEITH. 'Needling doubts about where to vaccinate'. *Br Med J* 1988, 297:779–80.

WEISS, R. AND THIER, S. O. 'HIV testing is the answer–what's the question'. *N Engl J Med* 1988, 319:1010–12.

WILSON, J. M. G. Personal communication, 1990.

Wofsy, C. B. 'Human immunodeficiency virus infection in women'. *JAMA* 1987, 257:2074–6.

WORLD HEALTH ORGANISATION. *Objectives of Youth Advisory Services.* Copenhagen, WHO Regional Office for Europe, 1977.

5 SCREENING IN ADULT MEN

In a man's middle years there is scarcely a
part of the body he would hesitate to turn
over to the proper authorities
(E. B. WHITE: *A Weekend with the Angels, 1954*)

INTRODUCTION

THERE IS SOUND EVIDENCE TO SUGGEST THAT PREVENTIVE
measures, and screening in particular, are most effective in the very young (D'Souza 1976). In the United
Kingdom with our system of primary care there are
excellent opportunities for using this fact to advantage
since most pregnant women and those with babies and
young children will have regular contact with the
health system through their general practitioner.

The position on screening in adults is more complex.
Our first approach was to consider screening in adult
men and women purely from an age point of view,
dividing the larger age range into two—young adulthood (25–44 years) and middle age (45–64 years).
Elegant as this might have been, it does not fit well with
reality. For practical reasons in this review we are,
therefore, regarding adulthood as covering the age
range 25 to 64 years and will consider men and women
separately. There will inevitably be a certain amount of
overlap and untidiness in the examples as, for instance,
with coronary heart disease which we will consider in
this chapter while recognising that it is a significant
health problem also and increasingly for women. We
consider psychiatric disease, particularly depression in
this chapter and diabetes in Chapter 6, although these
diseases obviously affect both sexes and other age
groups.

Early adulthood, particularly in men, tends to be a
period of low health service usage when health remains

fairly stable. With middle age, usage begins to increase as symptoms present and health education and promotion messages begin to appear more relevant. Table 14 shows the opportunities for health service contact in adult men.

TABLE 14. *Opportunities for health service contact in adult men*

LOCATION	TYPE OF HEALTH PROFESSIONAL
General practice	GP, health visitor, practice nurse
Hospital	Specialist medical or paramedical hospital staff as appropriate
Community	Dentist, chiropodist, optometrist, pharmacist
Work	Occupational health physician, company doctor

Traditionally, as we have already seen, screening in adults, as to a somewhat lesser extent in other age groups, has tended to be disease-oriented. Programmes have been set up to identify particular diseases, often before they have been subjected to evaluation and scientific scrutiny. In 1963 Wilson reviewed the concept of multiple screening and in the late 1960s and 1970s, several trials of multiphasic screening were carried out to see if general health screening in populations would improve health. Results of two such studies—one in the United States (Cutler *et al* 1973) and one in the United Kingdom (South East London Screening Study Group 1977)—failed to show any benefit in terms of either morbibity or mortality, and the concept of multi-phasic screening was largely discredited. There are of course numerous private and work-related schemes of multiple screening but evidence of their benefit is lacking.

The emphasis today remains very much on screening for specific conditions although increasing attention is also being paid to screening for risk factors for disease. But again caution in any advocacy of screening in this age group is essential. For many of the conditions which cause illness and death during this period of life we do have adequate methods of diagnosis. However in many too we lack an adequate knowledge of aetiology and, in conditions such as multiple sclerosis, arthritis, and motor neurone disease, an effective method of treatment. Screening in these conditions cannot therefore be justified. Similarly, chronic bronchitis and indeed respiratory disease in general are an important cause of morbidity and mortality but do not satisfy the criteria for screening.

The main causes of death in adult men are shown in Table 15. As the first part of the table shows, the two main causes of death in young adult men (25–44 years) are malignancies and external causes (including road accidents and suicide) with circulatory and heart disease coming a strong third. In middle age, circulatory disease takes precedence over malignant diseases. Screening efforts have thus far been concentrated overwhelmingly on coronary heart disease and its main risk factors and on carcinomas of various types. One area highlighted in Table 15 that certainly merits attention is mortality from external causes, including motor vehicle accidents and suicide.

In this chapter we shall consider briefly the question of screening for depression and then review the present position on screening for coronary heart disease and cancer in adult men with a brief look at occupational health screening which is relevant in this age group.

DEPRESSION

It may be that better methods of screening for psychiatric diseases, including depression, could help to identify those most at risk. Depression is one of the most common problems seen in general practice (Katon 1987) but, as Goldberg and Tantum (1990) point out, evidence that detection of psychiatric disturbance by screening test actually benefits the patient is hard to come by. A

TABLE 15. *Main causes of death in adult men (England and Wales 1986)*

CAUSE	NUMBER		% TOTAL DEATHS	
Young adulthood (25–44 years)				
Malignant diseases	1777		20	
External causes				
Motor vehicle accidents	828		9·3	
Suicide	1038	3065	11·7	34·5
Others	1199		13·5	
Circulatory disease				
IHD	1548	2281	17·4	25·7
Others	733		8·3	
Diseases of the nervous system including mental disorders	477		5·4	
Respiratory disease	325		3·7	
Other causes	946		10·7	
	8871		100	
Middle age (45–64 years)				
Circulatory disease				
Ischaemic heart disease	22523		38·8	
Other heart disease	1231	28828	2·1	49·7
Cerebrovascular disease	3329		5·7	
Others	1745		3·0	
Malignant disease				
Trachea, bronchus, lung	6836		11·8	
Alimentary tract	4671	18484	8·0	31·8
Others	6977		12·0	
Respiratory disease	3458		6·0	
Other causes	7237		12·5	
	58007		100	

study by Johnstone and Goldberg (1976) showed that treatment by the family doctor after detection of a psychiatric disorder by screening reduced the length of time those patients experienced symptoms by an average of 2·1 months compared to a control group and suggested that the effect was particularly marked in those with very high scores at first consultation. In another study patients with high scores on a depression questionnaire were randomised to treatment and no treatment groups. The treated group did very much better than the untreated (Zung et al 1983).

However, in a study by Hoeper and colleagues (1984), it appeared that doctors did not increase their rate of identification of psychiatric disorders as a result of information provided by a screening test. Shapiro and colleagues (1985) also randomised patients into a group whose doctors received feedback of scores on a screening questionnaire and a group where no feedback occurred. Detection of emotional problems was only slightly higher in the feedback group than among the controls. Goldberg and Tantum (1990) suggest that mere feedback of scores is not in itself of any value unless the doctors concerned are interested in the information and prepared to discuss possible implications with the patients.

The US Preventive Services Task Force (1989) does not recommend routine screening for depression in asymptomatic people. The Canadian Task Force (1979) equally found little evidence to support screening for affective disorders. Screening for depression is supported by some authors (Lancet 1986). However, others have reviewed the evidence and concluded that screening is not appropriate (Campbell 1987).

There is no convincing evidence that starting treatment in the early stages of depression has greater long-term effectiveness than intervention after the traditional symptoms of the disease appear (Campbell 1987; Kamerow 1987). Since spontaneous remission can be expected to occur in at least 50 per cent of patients, an improvement as the result of spontaneous remission could be wrongly attributed to the benefits of early intervention (Campbell 1987). Finally, because of the stigma that psychiatric referral unfortunately still carries, false-positive labelling is particularly undesirable.

Depression therefore is not at present a realistic candidate for formal screening. However, as the US Preventive Services Task Force (1989) has emphasised, we would certainly support the case for improving the awareness of depressive symptoms by general practitioners and those in primary care so that fewer cases of depression escape detection.

CORONARY HEART DISEASE

As Rose (1990) points out, in the twentieth century cardiovascular diseases have taken over from the infectious diseases of the nineteenth century as the dominant cause of death in adults in industrialised countries.

Coronary heart disease (CHD) is now the leading cause of death in the United Kingdom and the facts about it have been summarised recently by Waine (1989). In 1987 CHD resulted in the death of 180,000 people in the United Kingdom—that is 21 an hour, 3500 a week, and 15,000 a month—and it accounts for 30 per cent of deaths in men and 25 per cent in women. Although a large percentage of deaths from CHD occur in those aged over 65 years, the foundations of the disease are laid earlier in life where efforts to reduce its impact must begin. The disease also represents a significant economic cost to the nation—in 1981/2, for example, it was the cause of the loss of 30m working days, £940m in lost production, and £355m in treatment costs (National Forum for Coronary Heart Disease Prevention 1988). As Waine (1989) points out, if CHD were an infectious disease, it would have been declared an epidemic and action to try to control its spread would have been taken. Yet the government and large portions of the medical profession still lack a coherent strategy for prevention. This may be partly because it is by no means a clear-cut health problem and as such the responsibility of the Departments of Health—as a report from the National Audit Office (1989) points out, decisions taken on matters such as agricultural policy and tobacco duty 'profoundly influence the underlying causes of heart disease'.

It is generally agreed that the main medical arm of attack against this epidemic has to be based at the primary care level but while there is evidence that many general practitioners are interested in becoming involved in preventive activities and health education and promotion, relatively few of them appear to be currently involved in this in an active way (Waller and Morgan 1987). This may change gradually with the introduction of the new contract of service in April 1990 with its emphasis on health promotion (Health Departments of Great Britain 1989). But there is also a danger, which we refer to later in this chapter when considering cholesterol, in moving the emphasis and thus the responsibility from a national to a local level, and as Walker and Shaper (1990) have recently pointed out, prevention of coronary heart disease requires a national food policy designed for health.

The Government's programme for improving primary health care (Secretaries of State 1987) rightly lays much emphasis on the role of the whole primary health care team.

> The Government intends positively to encourage family doctors and primary health care teams to increase their contribution to the promotion of good health. These professional workers as well as dentists and pharmacists are in daily contact with large numbers of the public and represent the front line of health care; they are therefore very well placed to persuade individuals of the importance of protecting their health; of the simple steps needed to do so; and of accepting that prevention is indeed better than cure.

Thus stated, it sounds both simple and possible, and there is no doubt, as we have seen earlier, that people are both more aware of their health and more prepared to take responsibility for it than they were even two decades ago. But there is a world of difference between giving advice and it being taken, as there is between prescribing a drug and ensuring compliance, and there is as wide a range of ability and commitment in a primary health care team as in any other type of workforce. However, there have been in recent years attempts in various research groups and practices to carry out screening for those at risk of CHD. In 1986 Shaper and colleagues drew attention to the fact that, although a reduction in ischaemic heart disease in Britain would require changes in the nation's diet, smoking habits, blood pressure, and habits of exercise, there was also a short-term need to identify people at particularly high risk. In order to develop a useful measure of risk, 7735 men aged 40–59 years, randomly selected from practices in 24 towns in England, Wales and Scotland were examined between 1978 and 1980 and a questionnaire was administered by a research nurse. After five years the association between each factor considered and risk of ischaemic heart disease was calculated and a scoring system devised which used years of cigarette smoking, mean blood pressure, recall of ischaemic heart disease or diabetes mellitus diagnosed by a doctor, history of parental death from 'heart trouble', and the presence of current angina on a chest pain questionnaire. The top fifth of the score distribution identified 53 per cent of men who had a major heart attack within five years of initial screening. The addition of age, serum total cholesterol, and resting electro-cardiographic findings only slightly improved prediction with considerable increase in cost and effort of screening.

As a result of subsequent discussions, Shaper and colleagues (1987) have made various modifications to the scoring system, including the substitution of systolic for mean blood pressure, and suggest the possibility of three systems—full, intermediate, and basic—as shown in Table 16. In terms of yield of cases of heart attack within the five years after screening there is very little to choose between the full and intermediate systems in percentage of cases occurring among men in the top fifth of each score (59 and 58 per cent respectively). The ECG it seems adds little extra benefit and would complicate the actual screening procedure

TABLE 16. *Three systems for scoring the risk of a heart attack. The two electrocardiographic criteria are mutually excusive**

RISK FACTORS	SCORING SYSTEM		
	FULL	INTERMEDIATE	BASIC (GP)
Age (yrs)	+	−	−
Smoking (yrs)	+	+	+
Systolic BP (mmHg)	+	+	+
Cholesterol (mmol/l)	+	+	−
ECG-definite MI	+	−	−
ECG-ischaemia	+	−	−
Diagnosis of IHD	+	+	+
Current angina (Q)	+	+	+
Diagnosis of diabetes	+	+	+
Parental death from 'heart trouble'	+	+	+
% IHD 'cases' in top fifth of score	59	58	54

*Adapted from Shaper *et al* (1987) and reproduced by kind permission of the authors and publisher.

both in terms of administration and interpretation of results, as well as being considerably more expensive. The basic (GP) score could be determined for all men in the appropriate age range who attend their doctor for any reason and the initial assessment could be carried out by a practice nurse or assistant. Thus there is available a simple risk score screening system for use at the primary care level.

Jones and co-workers (1988) have developed a screening model in which people aged 25–55 years in a Swansea practice of around 10,000 patients can be screened in about two and a half months by a team of nurses in an effort to identify those at risk. Risk factors considered included obesity, blood pressure, blood cholesterol level, family history, use of alcohol and tobacco. Of those invited for screening, 62 per cent attended with the use of only one reminder letter. Non-attenders are being followed up as part of a further study. These workers demonstrated that 64 per cent of patients found to have a high blood cholesterol concentration showed a positive response to life-style counselling in a clinic run by a dietitian or health visitor and suggest that, even without an analysis of non-attenders, this made the screening programme worthwhile. A more common approach is to identify those at high risk during routine consultation. This approach has the advantage that it does not depend on the individual's response to an invitation to be screened or on his or her commitment to prevention. As Waller and Morgan (1988) point out, GP consultation rates are higher for manual workers who are at higher risk of cardiovascular disease but are less likely to regard preventive medicine as a priority. Opportunistic recording of at risk factors by a practice nurse has also been reported by Anggard and colleagues (1986). Patients between the ages of 20 and 59 years can be referred during a consultation or refer themselves and their cardiovascular risk score can then be assessed. Around 19 health centres use this screening technique, the data are processed by microcomputer, and an immediate assessment of risk is available at the time of the initial interview. A specially trained practice nurse performs the initial screening and is also responsible for follow-up and health advice. This would seem to be a crucial factor throughout the whole spectrum of screening activities. In the absence of one person responsible for the operation and for overall co-ordination in whatever field, it is all too easy for results to get overlooked and follow-up neglected.

The Oxford Project for the Prevention of Heart Attack and Stroke was established in 1982 following publication in 1981 of a report on the *Prevention of Arterial Disease in General Practice* (RCGP 1981) which concluded that

about half of all strokes and a quarter of deaths from coronary heart disease in people under 70 are probably preventable by the application of existing knowledge.

The initial study included three general practices provided with low-cost, low-technology support from a 'facilitator', paid from research funds, which were compared with control practices in respect of identification of major risk factors for cardiovascular disease in middle-aged patients. Patients attending for a routine consultation with their doctor were asked to make an appointment with a practice nurse for a health check, and this was compared with the ordinary consultations in the control practices. The facilitator helped the practices to develop the nurse's role (Fullard *et al* 1984, 1987).

Evidence from the control practices showed that improvements in recording blood pressure, smoking habits, and weight occurred spontaneously during the study. But with the introduction into intervention practices of a systematic case-finding approach in which practice nurses conducted health checks and were helped by the facilitator, the improvement was greater—blood pressure recording doubled, recording of smoking habits quadrupled, and recording of weight increased five-fold. The model appeared to offer free, acceptable health checks and advice to patients.

The results show that ascertainment of the main risk factors for CHD in primary care can be improved substantially with an opportunistic systematic approach using practice nurses. About 90 per cent of the population could be offered such screening within a five year period and this would combine both the mass and risk strategy approaches to screening. In the study only about 5 per cent of patients declined the health check. A facilitator can begin and maintain such a programme in several practices more quickly and effectively than individual practices could do without such support.

Throughout the United Kingdom about 70 facilitators have now been appointed to visit practices and set up changes in systems of recording cardiovascular risk factors (National Forum for CHD Prevention 1988).

However, doubt has been expressed about the whole concept of risk factors and about the effect of population interventions on morbidity and morality. McCormick and Skrabanek (1988) have suggested that there is no evidence to justify the considerable resources in terms of time and money devoted to interventions such as screening and have also pointed out that the interventions are not themselves harmless. They cite, for example, the results of the largest trial, the World Health Organisation collaborative trial (1986) which showed no difference in mortality from CHD between the control and the intervention groups (p=0·8) and no difference in overall mortality (p=0·4). Yet the authors claimed that

> these benefits are large enough to be of great public health importance ... but they do not achieve the conventional level of significance and therefore, by themselves, constitute only moderate evidence that intervention is effective. Thus 'it would appear that statistical evaluation can be disregarded, if it does not support a foregone conclusion' (McCormick and Skrabanek 1988).

Fries, Green and Levine (1989), however, suggest that these arguments, with their emphasis on mortality, embody the assumption that the sole purpose of health promotion is life extension. In their opinion, the main purpose of most health promotion activities in developed societies is to improve the quality of life, to compress morbidity, and to extend active life expectancy. They also make the point that in our kind of society, with the dramatic improvements in life expectancy seen this century, overall total mortality rates are becoming stubbornly resistant to either preventive or curative interventions.

Gunning-Schepers and colleagues from Rotterdam (1989) also point out that, although McCormick and Skrabanek may ultimately prove to be right, there is as yet insufficient evidence to stop the advice to the population to stop smoking, limit their fat intake, and know their blood pressure. When medication is contemplated, on the other hand, costs and benefits should be very carefully evaluated.

Three Main Risk Factors for CHD

The three main risk factors for CHD are cigarette smoking, hypertension, and raised blood cholesterol concentration, with the subsidiary factors of positive family history and overweight.

Cigarette smoking

The simple question 'do you smoke?' is certainly the cheapest and possibly the most effective form of screening for risk of CHD, as for many other diseases such as chronic bronchitis and cancer of the lung. The young adult age group is, as we have said, generally healthy but it is also a stage of life at which many people embark on life-time habits that can be seriously damaging to health (D'Souza 1976). The most important of these is cigarette smoking and, as Russell and colleagues (1979) have shown, one year after receiving advice from their GP to stop smoking, re-inforced by a leaflet and with notice of follow-up, 5 per cent of patients had ceased to smoke. Evidence from the Oxford Project suggests that advice from doctors on this point is more likely to be heeded than that given by nurses.

The US Preventive Services Task Force (1989) recommend that tobacco cessation counselling should be offered on a regular basis to all patients who smoke and that adolescents and young adults who do not smoke should be positively advised not to start.

About half of the cigarette smoker's excess mortality is due to cardiovascular disease (Rose 1990) and in nearly all studies cigarette smoking has emerged as a major risk factor for coronary heart disease, with a relative risk as high as five among younger men (Doll and Peto 1977) but fallng with age. In contrast the attributable risk is high at all ages in both sexes. The coronary mortality rates of those who give up smoking are much lower than the rates of those who continue to smoke (Doll and Peto 1977, Rose et al 1982).

High blood pressure

As with questions about smoking, there is little controversy in the measurement of hypertension as a preventive screening measure in primary care. It is one of the best predictors of risk for CHD with systolic pressure being marginally better than diastolic (Rose 1987). The US Preventive Services Task Force (1989) recommended that blood pressure should be measured regularly in all persons aged 3 years and over. The Canadian Task Force (1984) suggested that all those aged over 25 years should have their blood pressure measured during any visit to a physician. In the United Kingdom there is no national policy although the 1990 contract for general practice in the National Health Service (Health Departments of Great Britain 1989) does include a new sessional fee for health promotion clinics including those designed to cover risk factors for heart disease.

The measurement of blood pressure is a straightforward procedure and can be easily incorporated into a routine consultation with a general practitioner or carried out by a practice nurse. Results of studies in the United States (Veterans Administration Cooperative Study Group 1967, 1970; Hypertension Detection and Follow-up Program Co-operative Group 1979), Australia (Management Committee 1980), and Britain (Medical Research Council 1977, 1985) have suggested that controlling raised blood pressure is effective in reducing risk of stroke and may be so in the case of CHD. However further evaluation studies are needed. Satisfactory methods of treatment of blood pressure are available—they are effective and have few side-effects.

The North Karelia Project set up in Finland in 1972 in an effort to control and reduce cardiovascular diseases (Puska, Tuomilehto and Salonen 1981; Puska, Salonen and Nissinen 1983) included the establishment of special hypertension clinics run by public health nurses to improve opportunistic case-finding and facilitate control and follow-up of patients on anti-hypertensive therapy. In the first few years of the project special mass screening sessions for hypertension were organised. Within five years it became clear that mass screening yields of new individuals with hypertension had diminished markedly and the emphasis changed to opportunistic case-finding as the screening method of choice. Based on this experience the national plan prepared in Finland for the detection, treatment and follow-up of subjects with hypertension did not recommend widespread mass screening but favoured an intensification of case-finding within the framework of existing health services.

In a recent cost-effectiveness analysis study, Edgar and Schnieden (1989) constructed two hypothetical programmes aimed to detect and treat mild hypertension in residents of Stockport District Health Authority. The first programme involved population screening, the second an opportunistic case-finding exercise in general practice. Their results favoured the second approach for a number of reasons.

Firstly, given conditions approaching full take-up, case-finding is more cost-effective in total and health service costs.

Secondly, population screening carries with it the implicit undertaking that those who volunteer for the programme will derive benefit. Treatment of mild hypertension is associated with only a marginal improvement in the individual risk of developing a stroke and can not be said unequivocally to meet the benefit condition. Indeed, as Skrabanek and McCormick (1989) point out, the results of the Medical Research Council Trial of treating patients with mild to moderate hypertension with either propranolol or bendrofluazide against placebo showed no benefit in reduction of all cause mortality in those who had received active treatment (MRC 1985).

Thirdly, compliance with treatment is also very important and this will vary from individual to individual for a variety of reasons. This may be more adequately assessed and controlled in the general practice setting in consultation between the doctor and his patient than in the less personal screening session. Finally, there is a problem of differential take-up of invitations to screening. By taking the opportunity to examine the blood pressure of patients as they see their general practitioners, it is estimated that over 90 per cent of the population can be tested in a five-year period and that this approach is likely to reach subjects from all social groups. Although there remain social inequalities in health, these do not seem to apply to access to primary care (Collins and Klein 1980). However, Edgar and Schnieden (1989) caution that establishment of such case-finding programmes will require fairly fundamental change at primary care level. There is still wide variation between doctors committed to health prevention and promotion who succeeded in case-finding programmes (Barber *et al* 1979; Hall 1985) and those who have failed to take advantage of opportunities provided by routine consultation (Heller and Rose 1977; Michael 1984). There is also the ever-present spectre of records systems. Without a fundamental change in the records systems still in use in many practices, implementation of case-finding programmes would be extremely difficult to evaluate and monitor (Coope 1984).

Cholesterol

Cholesterol testing is a prime current example of the continuing controversy in screening between the enthusiasts and the sceptics.

In the United States there is a high public awareness of the significance of cholesterol and overwhelming demand for mass screening services but, as in this country, there remains a division of opinion on the value of this. In 1984 the National Institutes of Health convened a Consensus Development Conference on Lowering Blood Cholesterol to Prevent Heart Disease (National Cholesterol Education Program 1987). They recommended that individuals with blood cholesterol levels above the 75th percentile of the US cholesterol distribution be treated intensively to lower their cholesterol level, thus defining a quarter of the US adult population as being at sufficiently increased risk to warrant intensive intervention. In 1985, the National Heart Lung and Blood Institute (NHLBI) launched the National Cholesterol Education Program (NCEP 1988), a nationwide effort to reduce the prevalence of high blood cholesterol through education of professionals and the public. It has also funded three projects to explore the feasibility of various public screening strategies and of developing methods of education and channels of referral to ensure that those identified receive appropriate care and advice.

However, despite the enthusiasm for public screening, the National Cholesterol Education Program members (1987) admit that current knowledge of certain elements which will affect the success of screening programmes is inadequate. These elements include the willingness and ability of primary care physicans to deal with large numbers of referrals, the reliability of measurements, and how to encourage compliance of those screened with the advice they receive. They conclude that further information is needed and failure to pay attention to these issues could significantly reduce the effectiveness of public screening programmes.

The importance of the follow-up point is emphasised in a report from the Minnesota Heart Health Program (Rastam et al., 1988a). During a one-year period 424 adults from a population-based screening and education programme were referred to medical care after twice having raised levels of blood cholesterol. Two hundred and eighty (66 per cent) reported substantial dietary change, either self-initiated or as a result of seeing a doctor. Nineteen subjects (5 per cent) were on lipid-lowering drugs. However, one-third had not sought medical or other appropriate advice. In another report from the same programme, Rastam and colleagues (1988b) point out that the proposed cut-off levels for referral will yield a large number of people requiring follow-up advice and treatment. It is essential, and by no means a foregone conclusion, that resources to do this adequately are available before mass screening programmes are started.

The US Preventive Services Task Force (1989) recommended periodic measurement of total serum cholesterol for middle-aged men and note that this may also be clinically prudent in young men, women, and the elderly. All patients should also receive periodic counselling on dietary intake of fat. Their report states that serum cholesterol testing in the United States has the potential to achieve a significant reduction in the nationwide incidence of coronary artery disease. However, the Task Force also cautions that care is essential to guard against unnecessary health care expenditure and adverse personal consequences.

In particular, the use of inaccurate laboratory or desktop instruments for screening can lead to large numbers of both false-negative and false-positive results. The former can delay needed clinical intervention and the latter can lead to considerable inconvenience, costs, and adverse psychological and medical consequences in persons not needing intervention.

In the United Kingdom too there is a division of opinion on the value of screening for blood cholesterol. The Coronary Prevention Group has called for the introduction of cholesterol testing as part of a comprehensive strategy to prevent CHD (BMJ, 1989).

The Group recommends three stages to the process of general screening. First, assessment by general practitioners of risk factors for all patients, and the provision of information on how to reduce their risk. Secondly, measurement of cholesterol in those identified as being at high risk, with advice on diet and lifestyle as a first line of attack and drug treatment as a second if cholesterol levels fail to respond to changes in behaviour. Thirdly, cholesterol testing and relevant advice on risk reduction should be extended to all patients.

In July 1988, the Secretary of State for Health announced that he had invited the Standing Medical Advisory Committee

> to consider whether opportunistic cholesterol testing can make a cost-effective contribution towards identifying and treating people at increased risk of coronary heart disease.

In our view it is vital that cholesterol testing does not prove to be another example of a universal screening programme becoming politically expedient before it has been scientifically evaluated. Shaper (1989) in a comment on the National Audit Office report on CHD emphasises the point that, while widespread blood cholesterol measurement may appear to be a move towards the control and prevention of CHD, it is far more likely to promote the use of lipid-lowering drugs which are costly, as yet of unknown long-term safety, and unproved in women. Shaper also draws attention to the danger that the focus on primary care as an excellent situation for screening and identification of high-risk subjects would transfer much of the responsibility for the CHD problem from central government to the local level. A major population strategy is also essential in terms, for example, of health education, food and agricultural policy, provision of exercise facilities, and fiscal and advertising policies on tobacco. He concludes

> the burden of this comment is to make it clear that government should not be allowed to avoid major responsibility for action against CHD by minor activity in the field of primary care.

Walker and Shaper (1990) also point out that, while there is no doubt that blood cholesterol is an essential factor in CHD, the question of how useful it is for predicting heart attack in populations where many have a high blood cholesterol level remains open.

One of the issues of concern in this country, as in the United States, centres on the resources available to deal with the level of referrals and the quality of those resources. One recent study was carried out to obtain information on the dietary knowledge of primary health care workers and on their ability to apply this knowledge in practice (Francis et al 1989). One hundred and twenty-eight primary health care workers (53 GPs and 61 nurses) in 12 practices and 14 primary care facilitators were surveyed by questionnaire between December 1987 and June 1988 on issues related to managing patients with moderate hypercholesterolaemia. All the practices were involved in a project to promote prevention in primary care and offered health checks to identify and deal with cardiovascular risk factors. They could thus have been reasonably expected to be above average with regard to motivation and knowledge. The results of the study, however, revealed gaps in knowledge and in ability to give practical, appropriate and positive dietary advice. An earlier study of GPs in London produced similar results (Avenell, Treherz and Tompkins 1985). It is clearly essential that adequate follow-up and counselling services by properly informed professionals are available.

Quality control of measurements is another aspect of concern and a recent study has addressed this (Broughton, Bullock and Cramb 1989). Three surveys were made of the quality of plasma cholesterol measurements performed with a commercial desk top analyser in primary care. In each survey some participants consistently failed to obtain results which agreed with the majority. The most common causes of error appeared to be poor technique and the use of time-expired re-agent strips. Broughton and colleagues (1989) state that users of such tests outside the laboratory require training and they suggest some simple guidelines which include contact with a local clincial chemistry laboratory for training and support and participation in external quality assessment schemes.

It is also the case that cholesterol concentrations are almost universally too high in Britain (Tunstall-Pedoe et al 1989), and that change of diet rather than giving drugs should be the preferred method of treatment (Study Group, European Atherosclerosis Society 1988). A recent review (Leitch, 1989) of reports on measuring cholesterol in the United Kingdom revealed that there appears to be no national consensus among experts as to who should be screened. An editorial in the *Lancet* (Tunstall-Pedoe 1989) acknowledges that patients will increasingly expect to know their cholesterol concentrations and GPs will therefore have to become better at assessing risk factors, counselling and giving dietary advice.

> They will also need to defuse the panic caused by simplistic artithmetical interpretation of meretricious, isolated cholesterol tests.

Selective testing, using clinical judgment, is more rational and cost-effective than mass screening and is the policy of choice at present in Britain today.

As was the case with screening for cervical cancer, screening programmes are often started prematurely and are then very difficult to stop or control (Smith *et al* 1989). Some health authorities and many general practitioners have already started population screening of blood cholesterol level and it is essential, before there is any further expansion of screening, that there is a critical review of the evidence. As Smith and colleagues (1989) emphasise, screening programmes in which doctors approach apparently healthy people and make them lifelong patients must, from an ethical as well as a human point of view, be sure that treatment facilities are available, that treatment is of proven efficacy, and that it does more good than harm. These requirements cannot yet be satisfied in the case of screening for cholesterol.

Brett (1989) makes the additional important point that the private exchange between the patient and the general practitioner is rarely examined in detail when the results of large drug trials are discussed 'yet it is at this encounter that most clinical decisions are made'. He also suggests that investigators understandably cast the results of years of research in the most optimistic light and continues

> however, a strongly interventionist perspective colors the published findings of the large trials of lipid-lowering drugs that have involved asymptomatic persons. Physicians must recognise this perspective before extrapolating from the clinical studies to office practice.

This is sound advice. Responsible clinical decision-making for individual patients ought to reflect both the possibilities and the limitations of the published data.

SO SHOULD WE SCREEN FOR RISK OF CORONARY HEART DISEASE?

The current position on Screening for Risk of Coronary Heart Disease is covered in a report of a Workshop on that subject (Oliver, Ashley-Miller, and Wood 1987). As Sir John Reid, then Chief Medical Officer at the Scottish Home and Health Department, pointed out in his opening remarks,

> screening for 'risk' of a disease—particularly where that risk is being quantified from the general experience of a population rather than specific individuals, and without the statistical precision that applies in many genetically determined diseases—raises new issues which call for careful consideration.

He states that, in coronary heart disease, there are really three main issues:

> whether, how and when to screen; the provision of advice to those "detected" (whatever that means); and the benefit/yield in terms of cost—this last being partly determined by the persuasiveness of the counsellor and the individual reaction to the advice which is proffered.

Oliver (1987), in a discussion of the problems and limitations of a mass screening strategy, asks the very proper question what do we tell those identifed as having raised cholesterol concentrations and raised blood pressure between the 50th and the 80th percentile? Their risk of CHD is only slightly increased, prediction of CHD is weak and cannot be individualised, and mass intervention thus far has been disappointing in its outcome. He challenges those who support mass screening programmes for the male adult population to ask themselves what they will do when screening identifies an otherwise fit, non-obese, 35-year-old man with serum cholesterol or blood pressure in the sixth or seventh deciles. Should he be told? If so, what should he be told about his individual risk and how to reduce it? Should the test be repeated in one or five years' time, or should the mildly abnormal result simply be noted and ignored?

In a session entitled 'Is Screening Needed?' a cardiologist, an epidemiologist, and a general practitioner gave their views, which despite some difference of emphasis, probably represent a reasonable consensus (de Bono, Shaper and Barber 1987). The cardiologist (de Bono) stated that screening has to be seen in the context of total care including health education and active treatment of established disease. For our population at the present time health education should have a higher priority than screening. He concludes

> in populations which already have an established healthy lifestyle and enjoy a high standard of medical care then preventive screening of high-risk groups is both logical and likely to be effective.

The epidemiologist (Shaper) felt that whole population screening for the identification of risk factors had little to recommend it. We already know that we are a population at high risk and we already know about the distribution and relative importance of the various risk factors. Identification of high-risk groups in whom intervention is likely to be effective and compliance high, can be carried out on an opportunistic basis in general practice by assessing the GP risk score for all middle-aged males who consult for any reason. This case-finding approach can be complemented by health education for the whole population.

The general practitioner (Barber) saw case-finding as a more practical approach than mass screening and one which could expect to cover the target population over a five-year period. However, he reminds that this required doctor motivation and runs the risk of excessive workload. It must therefore be a properly planned strategy and adequate and specially prepared record systems are essential for case-finding, management, and outcome review.

In summary, there is no current national policy on screening for risk of coronary heart disease in Britain and the position varies from area to area and from practice to practice.

CANCER

As Elwood (1985) has pointed out, the word cancer evokes for most of us a frightening picture of a relentlessly spreading disease. For this reason the concept that the earlier the disease is diagnosed the better, is an appealing one which carries with it the assumption that then it can be dealt with. Behind this attractively simple idea lies a screening minefield. If a test is to be used for the early detection of cancer, it has to fulfil some extremely strict criteria. It must be capable of detecting tumours before they cause symptoms. It must be very accurate to avoid the erroneous re-assurance and unjustified anguish of both false-negative and false-positive results. Ideally, since it will be widely applied, it must be inexpensive, safe and acceptable to the public. And even if such a test exists for a specific type of cancer, it must also be proved that earlier diagnosis will lead to treatment and that the treatment will be effective. There are tumours which even at an early stage do not respond well to treatment and there are tumours, such as non-melanoma skin cancers, for which treatment is so successful that slightly earlier diagnosis is not going to produce any marked improvement. It thus seems wise, as Chamberlain (1983) has pointed out, to limit screening services to those types of tumour where there is definite evidence of benefit.

If we look at the ranking of cancer screening programmes in order of the scientific evidence available on their effectiveness, the position is clear and simple. At the top of the list come cancer of the breast and cancer of the cervix which we will consider in the next chapter on adult women. Next come colorectal cancer or cancer of the large bowel, which affects both sexes equally but which we will consider in this chapter, and cancer of the lung. There are other tumours for which screening tests are available but they are not relevant to the general population of this country. Thus screening for gastric cancer seems to be a useful technique in Japan where this is the leading form of cancer and where some of the recent decrease in mortality may be attributable to the effect of the nationwide early detection programme (Hirayama *et al* 1985) but is not appropriate in the British population. Occupational screening for cancer of the bladder will be considered in the section on occupational screening at the end of the chapter.

Colorectal cancer

Colorectal cancer is an important health problem in this country in terms of morbidity and mortality and is second of the cancers in frequency to lung cancer in men and breast cancer in women (Chamberlain 1983). There is evidence that colorectal cancer arises primarily from pre-malignant adenomas and that the lead time from the benign lesion to invasive cancer is several years (Winawer and Miller 1987). It should therefore be possible to reduce mortality by a secondary prevention programme and two screening tests have been extensively evaluated. The faecal occult blood test has a good predictive value for neoplasia in patients aged 50 years and over. The stage of detected cancers is favourable for treatment and survival prospects are good. More than half of patients with positive tests, however, will have no evidence of benign or malignant neoplasia in the colon or rectum, and no more than 15–16 per cent of patients with a positive test will have cancer (Winawer and Miller 1987). Proctosigmoidoscopy is the other main screening procedure but it is an unpleasant test from the patient's point of view and there are no data available to estimate its sensitivity and specificity.

Opinions on whether or not to screen for colorectal cancer are mixed. The US Preventive Services Task Force (1989) stated that there is insufficient evidence to make a recommendation for or against faecal occult blood testing or sigmoidoscopy as effective population screening tests. However they suggest that this type of screening should be continued where it is already practised and should be available to those who request it. They also suggest that it may be 'clinically prudent' to offer screening to those aged 50 years and over with known risk factors for colorectal cancer.

In a series of three articles on occult blood screening, Frank (1985 a,b,c) concludes that more evidence is needed of the test's efficacy, effectiveness, and efficiency before it can be recommended for routine health maintenance in any age-group. He maintains that because of its low positive predictive value for cancer, the risky and expensive investigations necessary to confirm a possible diagnosis, and its questionable sensitivity, there must be considerable doubt as to whether the test does more good than harm. Until good experimental evidence is available of the test's ability to produce significant reductions in mortality at reasonable cost, its routine application to asymptomatic patients 'represents premature enthusiasm rather than thoughtful medical practice'.

A feasiblity study in general practice (Hardcastle et al 1983) showed promising results in terms of yield of early cancer and adenomatous polyps and in the sensitivity and specificity of the faecal occult blood test. And in another study in general practice, Lallemand and colleagues (1984) suggested that, in view of the magnitude of the problem and the long lead time, it is reasonable to seek to improve outcome by trying to identify pre-symptomatic patients. However, a randomised trial of compliance with screening for colorectal cancer in 14 general practices (Nichols *et al* 1986) produced no firm evidence that premature mortality could be reduced by screening for the disease and suggested that most general practitioners are not at the moment in favour of such screening.

Four large controlled trials to evaluate the faecal occult blood test with or without routine proctosigmoidoscopy are in progress—two in the United States, one in England and one in Sweden. Preliminary results from the Nottingham study (Hardcastle *et al* 1989) suggest that cancers detected by screening were at a less advanced pathological stage than those appearing in a control population. However, these authors emphasise that it is still too early to show any effect of screening on mortality from colorectal cancer and that the institution of a national population screening service, based on faecal occult blood tests, cannot be recommended until mortality rates are shown to decline. This seems a most sensible conclusion.

Lung cancer

Lung cancer has been studied extensively from the point of view of screening and illustrates very well one of the dilemmas that screening poses. There are effective screening tests which can detect early cases of lung cancer—regular chest X-rays together with sputum cytology can detect early tumours. However, such early detection has not been shown to improve mortality— these 'early' tumours are still relatively advanced and available treatment is not very effective (Elwood 1985, Fontana and Taylor 1978). The net result of screening, therefore, seems to be to inform patients earlier that they have a fatal disease and subject them to radical surgery which does not cure them (Chamberlain 1983).

There is general agreement that current evidence does not support routine population screening for lung cancer (US Preventive Services Task Force 1989, Morrison in press).

In the United States, where lung cancer is the leading cause of cancer death for both men and women, there have been suggestions that the possibility of screening in people aged over 65 years should be explored. In a study of age trends of lung cancer stage at diagnosis, O'Rourke and colleagues (1987) found that a group aged 65 years and over was at greater risk for lung cancer and had a higher proportion of lung cancer initially seen at local stage than younger groups. They comment that the American Cancer Society does not recommend screening for early detection of cancer of the lung and state

> we do not disagree with a policy that rejects mass screening for lung cancer... We would recommend, however, study of the efficacy of selective screening of target groups who are at particularly high risk for more localized lung cancer.

At present, therefore, as Greenwald and Cullen (1985) have stressed, the most desirable approach for reducing mortality from lung cancer continues to be a reduction in cigarette smoking. The most effective method of screening for risk of lung cancer, as well as chronic bronchitis and other respiratory diseases, would be the simple question—do you smoke cigarettes?—in the course of a routine consultation with a general practitioner.

OCCUPATIONAL SCREENING

Occupational screening differs from general health screening in that it usually takes place outside the normal routine health care provided by the National Health Service and is a specialised area of public health where groups of different background and ages are exposed to similar conditions. It is a very complex field and one that we do not attempt to cover in any detail in this book. However, particularly in adulthood, it is an important and valid part of the total health care of many individuals and should be included in this context.

Screening in the occupational setting can take place at three main levels. The first, particularly prominent in the United States, is worksite screening or health promotion with voluntary screening services and general health promotion packages available to employees. Johnson and Johnson are among firms which have been particularly active in this field in the United States with their 'Live for Life' programme of health status assessment. Firm evidence is still lacking on the effectiveness of this type of approach although those in favour claim that worksite health promotion not only increases productivity but decreases medical insurance costs.

However, in a recent evaluation of a worksite programme for the modification of cardiovascular risk factors in Australia Edye and colleagues (1989) suggest that individual health counselling was not effective in the long-term modification of mildly raised cardiovascular risk factors. They carried out a randomised controlled trial in volunteers working for Australian government organisations with follow-up three years later. Results indicated that a programme of individual counselling by occupational-health personnel at the worksite, which was directed at the improvement of risk factors for coronary heart disease, did not achieve major long-term improvements. However, the intervention appeared to have had some small effect on systolic blood pressure in men who were aged 40 years or over or in men employed in the administrative category. They conclude that individual counselling at the worksite in the form that was evaluated in the study appears to be of limited value in reducing cardiovascular risk factors and suggest that resources would be better used in campaigns to alter risk factors in the community as a whole.

The second level for occupational screening, which is becoming more common, is pre-employment screening. The form this takes can vary from a simple self-completed questionnaire—a superficial device designed mainly to protect an employer should a serious chronic health problem not declared subsequently manifest itself—to a very detailed medical examination and tests undergone, for example, by those seeking to work offshore in the North Sea. There are two main problems associated with this type of screening. The first concerns the need to assess constantly whether the screening required for a particular kind of employment remains relevant. One example of this is the routine pre-employment chest X-ray examination for NHS employees which was recently scrutinised by Jachuck and colleagues (1988). In 1978, to minimise cost and prevent unnecessary radiation, the Department of Health and Social Security issued guidelines which recommended radiological screening only for a selected group of NHS employees at risk of contracting tuberculosis at work. However, the test is not mandatory and it seems that not all employees thought to be at risk are offered screening (Jachuck and Bound 1983; BMJ Editorial 1984), despite the British Thoracic Society's recommendations that all immigrants from high-risk countries should be screened (Joint Tuberculous Committee of the British Thoracic Society 1983). On the basis of recent experience., Jachuck and colleagues (1988) suggest that evidence of BCG vaccination and the tuberculin skin test should be used to screen all NHS employees to control tuberculosis with chest X ray for those who cannot produce such evidence or show specified grades of Heaf reaction.

The second problem is that minor defects may be found that will unfairly and unnecessarily exclude someone from employment. While screening in this context is extremely specialised and takes place for a specific purpose and outside the normal remit of health care, these two points are certainly of importance in screening in general. The relevance of screening tests must be constantly evaluated to make sure firstly that they are necessary and secondly that they are measuring what they are meant to measure. And it is essential also to be aware of the possible fall-out from screening—that is, that what is found can be dealt with and not merely identified leaving individuals with an insoluble problem they did not previously know they had and labelled as ill, with possible implications for employment, insurance and other important factors.

The third and main level for occupational screening is screening for specific occupational hazards—for example, chest X-rays for coalminers and others working in dusty environments; regular tests for those working with lead, asbestos, and other potentially harmful substances. Unlike the other two strands of occupational screening, this is a statutory obligation on employers. From 1 October 1989 in Britain regulations on the Control of Substances Hazardous to Health (COSHH regulations) placed an added legal obligation on employers to assess the potential health risks created by work with hazardous substances and obliged them to establish guidelines and form a code of practice to reduce or even eliminate risk. As Seaton (1989) has pointed out, these new regulations come at a time when the public is increasingly aware of industrial hazards and they provide a potential framework for preventive action. However, enforcement requires that they are understood by all employers and that the Health and Safety Executive can oversee their implementation. This will not be easy, especially perhaps in smaller companies whose safety practices may be less well developed in the first place.

Occupational hazards are among the known causes of cancer which are subject to regulatory control and thus especially suitable for prevention. The perception exists that when specific carcinogenic agents are identified in the occupational environment they can be controlled and this contrasts with aspects of lifestyle, such as smoking and diet, where control requires a modification of cultural and personal behaviour patterns. Merletti and Segnan (1988) draw attention to the fact that personal choice plays little or no part in occupational exposure in the way that cigarette smokers, for example, can reduce their risk of contracting lung cancer by giving up the habit, and it is therefore important that maximum attention is paid to the safety of industrial processes. Equally, screening cannot be relied on as an occupational cancer control activity. As Merletti and Segnan (1988) also emphasise, there is no real evidence that screening for occupationally-induced cancer brings about any benefit. If screening is carried out in this context, it should only be done under circumstances where its effects can be evaluated.

An example of occupational screening at this level which is relevant to adult men is screening for cancer of the bladder, one of the 10 most common male cancers in Britain.

Bladder cancer

Screening for cancer of the bladder has been in operation in Britain since the 1950s. At the present time screening takes place in the dye manufacturing and rubber industries (Parkes 1971, 1975; Cartwright 1985). The larger firms support their own laboratories, the smaller ones contribute to the few National Health Service laboratories that specialise in the techniques. All programmes will screen workers regularly (every 6 to 12 months) for life but, despite their backing by both unions and management, the overall uptake is rarely regular or greater than 60 per cent of the workforce.

A critical assessment of the value of bladder screening has yet to be made (Cartwright 1985). Maligant cell cytology (MCC) is the method of choice and the general lack of critical evaluation is unfortunate since screening by MCC has been carried for many years. However, it is obviously a sensitive industrial issue and most screening has been done by private programmes with little regard for the size of the screened population and subject to confidentiality in regard to results. There is also a lack of data about the outcome in patients identified who would naturally be referred to various different urologists, some of them in private practice. Cartwright and colleagues (1981) examined survival from cases identified in a dye-manufacturing company and matched non-industrial cases in Manchester. Screened chemical workers, screened non-industrial workers, and those not screened were included in the design of the study. The results showed lead-time bias and a 'debatable amount of true increase in survival in the screened group'.

The future of MCC screening will depend first on the identification of new groups at high risk from occupational contact with either traditional substances or new materials. Non-occupational high-risk groups may also exist—those exposed to cyclophosphamide, for example, or coarse fishermen who stain their maggots with powdered azo dyes (Cartwright et al 1983; Cartwright 1985). The future of such screening depends secondly on the availability of automated methods of screening, for instance, flow cytometry, that remove the observer biases from current methods. A third future priority should be the demonstration of effective methods of treating very early bladder disease—techniques such as intravesical chemotherapy are still being evaluated and should be an essential part of any screening scheme.

Early results of a study to test the theory that early detection plus treatment of the urothelium might modify the natural history of bladder cancer (Cartwright 1986) are promising for this approach. However re-assessment of risk groups and further and broader based evaluation is essential, and the possibility of screening the general population is unlikely to be of relevance in most circumstances.

This brief discussion of occupational screening does highlight three main problems applicable to screening in general which appear of particular relevance in terms of employment. The first of these is that of identifying a condition for which there is no effective treatment or which is actually irrelevant to the functioning of the individual but which will label them has having a condition or disease. The second is that of the relevance of tests which should be regularly reviewed, a point made earlier in the context of developmental screening in childhood. Thirdly, there is the difficulty of management of data obtained and the evaluation of screening tests. This is particularly so when screening takes place outside the normal health care framework. But it cannot be overemphasised that evaluation is fundamental to the practice of screening wherever performed.

SUMMARY AND CONCLUSIONS

Screening in adult men is not an area where there are any overwhelming candidates for mass population screening and there is at the present time no national policy on screening for any particular condition.

The 1990 contract for general practitioners (Health Departments of Great Britain 1989) emphasises that health promotion and the prevention of illness are an integral part of general medical services and should be provided for patients between the ages of 16 and 74 years either during routine consultation or in special sessions for those who have not consulted in the previous three years. Health promotion services expected include measurement of height, weight, and blood pressure, a simple urine analysis, and enquiry about lifestyle, use of alcohol and tobacco, exercise and diet. The rationale for including measurement of height and urine analysis is not clear.

Common screening practice for adult men at the moment, therefore, appears to favour opportunistic screening during routine consultations with a general practitioner for risk factors for cardiovascular and other diseases with advice on lifestyle and its effects on health as appropriate. This does seem to us to be the most sensible approach, implying as it does a gradual change of emphasis from secondary to primary prevention. However, as we have mentioned elsewhere, the implications for general practice, particularly in terms of workload, must be monitored carefully.

With regard specifically to coronary heart disease we would suggest that this huge health problem needs to be tackled at three levels. First, we would support the present approach of opportunistic screening in routine general practice consultation rather than population screening. However, it is essential that we address and answer scientifically questions on the benefit or harm of treating mild to moderate hypertension and the possible consequences of labelling as hypertensive people who had hitherto considered themselves healthy. They are legitimate questions and deserve to be taken seriously. Attention must also be paid to national standards of quality control in the measurement of risk factors such as blood pressure and cholesterol, and to the availability of adequate follow-up treatment, advice, and supervision. Secondly, far more emphasis must be placed on primary preventive policies which in the long-term will surely be more effective than secondary prevention. Preventive efforts and health education must begin much earlier in life and must be available to all sections of the population. Finally, any successful programme of prevention for coronary heart disease must ultimately depend on national food, agriculture, and taxation policies, directed towards health rather than on simply transferring responsibility to primary medical care and 'blaming' the individuals.

REFERENCES

ANGGARD, E. E., LAND, J. M., LENIHAN, C. J., PACKARD, C. J., PERCY, M. J., RITCHIE, L. D. AND SHEPHERD, J. 'Prevention of cardiovascular disease in general practice: a proposed model.' Br Med J 1986, 293:177–80.

AVENELL, A., TREHERTZ, J. AND TOMPKINS, A. Family doctors' knowledge of nutrition and coronary heart desease prevention! Proceedings of the Thirteenth International Conference of Nutrition. Cambridge: Nutritian Society, 1985.

BARBER, J. H., BEEVERS, D. C., FIFE, R. et al. 'Blood pressure screening and supervision in general practice'. Br Med J 1979, 1:843–6.

BRETT, A. S. 'Treating hypercholesterolemia'. N Engl J Med 1989, 321:676–80.

BRITISH MEDICAL JOURNAL. 'Tuberculosis in hospital doctors'. Editorial. Br Med J 1984, 289:1327–8.

BRITISH MEDICAL JOURNAL. 'Coronary Prevention Group calls for cholesterol testing for all'. Br Med J 1989, 298:252.

BROUGHTON, P. M. G., BULLOCK, D. G. AND CRAMB, R. 'Quality of plasma cholesterol measurements in primary care' Br Med J 1989, 298:297–8.

CAMPBELL, T. L., 'Controversies in family medicine: why screening for mental health problems is not worthwhile in family practice'. *J Fam Pract* 1987, 25:184–7.

CANADIAN TASK FORCE ON THE PERIODIC HEALTH EXAMINATION. 'The periodic health examination'. *Can Med Assoc J* 1979, 121:1194–254.

CANADIAN TASK FORCE ON THE PERIODIC HEALTH EXAMINATION. 1984 update. *Can Med Assoc J* 1984, 130:2–15.

CARTWRIGHT, R. A. 'Screening workers exposed to suspect bladder carcinogens'. *J Occ Med* 1986, 28(10):1017–9.

CARTWRIGHT, R. A. 'Screening for Bladder Cancer'. In *Screening for Cancer*. New York and London: Academic Press, 1985.

CARTWRIGHT, R. A. 'Historical and modern epidemiological studies on populations exposed to N-substituted Aryl compounds'. *Environ Hlth Perspect* 1983, 49:13–19.

CARTWRIGHT, R. A., GADIAN, T., GARLAND, J. B. AND BERNARD, S. M. 'The influence of malignant cell cytology screening on the survival of industrial bladder cancer cases'. *J Epidemiol Comm Hlth* 1981, 35:35–8.

CHAMBERLAIN, JOCELYN. Editorial: 'Screening for Cancer'. *Community Medicine* 1983, 5:283–6.

COLLINS, E. AND KLEIN, R. 'Equity and the NHS: self-reported morbidity, access and primary care'. *Br Med J* 1980, 281:111–5.

Control of substances hazardous to health regulations 1988. Approved code of practice. London: HMSO, 1988.

COOPE, J. 'Hypertension in general practice: what is to be done?' *Br Med J* 1984, 288:906–8.

CUTLER, J. L., RAMCHARAN, S., FELDMAN, R., *et al.* 'Multiphasic checkup evaluation study: 1. Methods and population'. *Prev Med* 1973, 2:197–206.

D'SOUZA, M. F. 'A general review of established screening procedures'. *Health Bull* 1976, 181:54–7.

DOLL, R. AND PETO R. 'Mortality among doctors in different occupations'. *Br Med J* 1977, 1:1433–6.

EDGAR, M. A. AND SCHNIEDEN, H. 'The economics of mild hypertension programmes'. *Soc Sci Med* 1989, 28:221–2.

EDYE, B. V., MANDRYK, J. A., FROMMER, M. S., HEALEY, S. AND FERGUSON, D. A. 'Evaluation of a worksite programme for the modification of cardiovascular risk factors'. *Med J Aust* 1989, 150:574–81.

ELWOOD, J. 'Screening for Cancer'. In *Screening for Cancer*. New York and London: Academic Press, 1985.

EUROPEAN ATHEROSCLEROSIS STUDY GROUP. 'Strategy for Prevention of Coronary Heart Disease: a Policy Statement of the EAS'. *Eur Hlth J* 1987, 8:77–88.

EUROPEAN ATHEROSCLEROSIS STUDY GROUP. 'The Recognition and Management of Hyperlipidaemia in Adults. A Policy Statement of the EAS'. *Eur Hlth J* 1988, 9:571–600.

FRANCIS, J., ROCHE, M. MANT, D., JONES, L. AND FULLARD, E. 'Would primary health care workers give appropriate dietary advice after cholesterol screening?' *Br Med J* 1989, 298:1620–2.

FRANK, J. W. 'Occult-blood screening for colorectal carcinoma: the benefits'. *Am J Prev Med* 1985a, 1:3–9.

FRANK, J. W. 'Occult-blood screening for colorectal carcinoma: the risks.' *Am J Prev Med* 1985b, 1:25–32.

FRANK, J. W. 'Occult-blood screening for colorectal carcinoma: the yield and the costs'. *Am J Prev Med* 1985c, 1:18–24.

FRIES, J. F., GREEN, L. W. AND LEVINE, S. 'Health promotion and the compression of morbidity'. *Lancet* 1989, i:481–3.

FONTANA, R. S. AND TAYLOR, W. F. 'Screening for lung cancer: the Mayo Lung Project'. In: *Screening in Cancer*. A. B. MILLER (ed.). Geneva: UICC Technical Report Series 1978, 40:233–53.

FULLARD, E., FOWLER, G., AND GRAY, J. A. M. 'Facilitating prevention in primary care'. *Br Med J* 1984, 289:1585–7.

FULLARD, E., FOWLER, G. AND GRAY, J. A. M. 'Promoting prevention in primary care: controlled trial of low technology, low cost approach'. *Br Med J* 1987, 294:1080–2.

GOLDBERG, D. AND TANTUM, D. 'Public health impact of mental disorders'. In *Oxford Textbook of Public Health*. Second edition. W. W. HOLLAND, R. DETELS, AND G. KNOX (eds). Volume 3, Section G. 'Interventions in Public Health' Oxford: Oxford University Press, 1990.

GOLDBERG, D. AND BRIDGES, K. 'Screening for Psychiatric Illness in General Practice: the General Practitioner versus the Screening Questionnaire'. *J R Coll Gen Practit* 1987, 37:15–18.

GREENWALD, P. AND CULLEN, J. W. Editorial. 'The new emphasis in cancer control. *J Natl Cancer Inst* 1985, 74:543–51.

GUNNING-SCHEPERS, L. J., BARENDREGT, J. J. AND VAN DER MAAS, P. J. 'Population interventions reassessed'. *Lancet* 1989, i:479–81.

HALL, J. A. 'Audit of screening for hypertension in general practice'. *J R Coll Gen Practit* 1985, 35:243.

HARDCASTLE, J. D., FARRANDS, P. A., BALFOUR, T. W., CHAMBERLAIN, J., AMAR, S. S. AND SHELDON, M. J. 'Controlled trial of faecal occult blood testing in the detection of colorectal cancer'. *Lancet* 1983, 193, ii:1–4.

HARDCASTLE, J. D., CHAMBERLAIN, J., SHEFFIELD, J. *et al*. 'Randomised, controlled trial of faecal occult blood screening for colorectal cancer'. *Lancet* 1989, i:1160–4.

HEALTH DEPARTMENTS OF GREAT BRITAIN. *General Practice in the National Health Service. The 1990 Contract*. Health Departments of Great Britain. 1989.

HELLER, R. F. AND ROSE, G. 'Current management of hypertension in general practice'. *Br Med J* 1977, 2:1442–4.

HIRAYAMA, T., HISAMICHI, S., FUJIMOTO, I., OSHIMA, A. AND TOMINAGA, S. 'Screening for Gastric Cancer'. In *Screening for Cancer*. New York and London: Academic Press, 1985.

HOEPER, E. W., KESSLER, L. G., NYCZ, G. R., BURKE, J. D. Jr, AND PIERCE, W. E. 'The usefulness of screening for mental illness'. *Lancet* 1984, i:33–5.

HYPERTENSION DETECTION AND FOLLOW-UP PROGRAM CO-OPERATIVE GROUP. Five-year findings of the Hypertension Detection and Follow-up Program. 1. Reduction in mortality of persons with high blood pressure including mild hypertension'. *JAMA* 1979, 242:2562–71.

JACHUCK, S. J. AND BOUND, C. L. 'Control and prevention of tuberculosis'. *Br Med J* 1983, 287:1722–3.

JACHUCK, S. J., BOUND, C. L., JONES, C. E. AND BRYSON, M. 'Is a pre-employment chest radiograph necessary for NHS employees?' *Br Med J* 1988, 296: 1187–8.

JOHNSTONE, A. AND GOLDBERG, D. P. 'Psychiatric screening in general practice: a controlled trial'. *Lancet* 1976, i:605–8.

JOINT TUBERCULOSIS COMMITTEE OF THE BRITISH THORACIC SOCIETY. 'Control and prevention of tuberculosis; a code of practice'. *Br Med J* 1983, 287:1118–21.

JONES, A., DAVIES, D. H., DOVE, J. R., COLLINSON, M. A. AND BROWN, P. M. R. 'Identification and treatment of risk factors for coronary heart disease in general practice: a possible screening model.' *Br Med J* 1988, 296:1711–14.

KAMEROW, D. B. 'Controversies in family practice: is screening for mental health problems worthwhile?' *J Fam Pract* 1987, 25:181–4.

KATON, W. 'The epidemiology of depression in medical care. *Int J Psychiatr* 1987, 17:93–112.

LALLEMAND, R. C., VAKIL, P. A., PEARSON, P. AND BOX, V. 'Screening for asymptomatic bowel cancer in general practice'. *Br Med J* 1984, 288:29–32.

Lancet. 'Treatment of depression in medical patients' (Editorial). *Lancet,* 1986. ii:949–50.

LEITCH, D. 'Who should have their cholesterol concentration measured? What experts in the UK suggest'. *Br Med J* 1989, 298:1615–6.

LEITCH, D. AND BEDFORD, B. 'Cholesterol screening in general practice'. *J Roy Coll Gen Practit* 1988, 38:518–9.

MANAGEMENT COMMITTEE. 'The Australian therapeutic trial in mild hypertension'. *Lancet* 1980, i:1261–7.

MCCORMICK, J. AND SKRABANEK, P. 'Coronary heart disease is not preventable by population intervention'. *Lancet* 1988, ii:839–41.

MEDICAL RESEARCH COUNCIL COMMITTEE ON MILD TO MODERATE HYPERTENSION. Randomised controlled trial of treatment for mild hypertension: design and pilot study'. *Br Med J* 1977, 1:1437–40.

MEDICAL RESEARCH COUNCIL WORKING PARTY. 'MRC trial of treatment of hypertension principal results'. *Br Med J* 1985, 291:97–104.

MERLETTI, F. AND SEGNAN, N. 'Occupational cancers'. In *Elimination or*

Reduction of Diseases. ALAN J. SILMAN AND SHANE P. A.
ALLWRIGHT (eds). Oxford: Oxford University Press, 1988.

MICHAEL, G. 'Quality of care in managing hypertension by casefinding in North West London'. *Br Med J* 1984, 288:906–8.

MORRISON, B. 'Lung cancer: a report for the Canadian Task Force on the Periodic Health Examination'. *Can Med Assoc J*, in presss, 1990.

NATIONAL AUDIT OFFICE. *National Health Service: Coronary Heart Disease.* London: HMSO, 1989.

NATIONAL CHOLESTEROL EDUCATION PROGRAM. Office of Prevention, Education and Control. National Heart, Lung and Blood Institute. Public Screening for Measuring Blood Cholesterol—Issues for Special Concern. A Statement from the National Cholesterol Education Program. US Dept of Health and Human Services. 5 October 1987.

NATIONAL CHOLESTEROL EDUCATION PROGRAM. *Current Status of Blood Cholesterol Measurement in Clinical Laboratories in the United States.* A Report from the Laboratory Standardisation Panel of the National Cholesterol Education Program. US Department of Health and Human Services, 1988.

NATIONAL FORUM FOR CORONARY HEART DISEASE PREVENTION. *Coronary Heart Disease Prevention: Action in the UK 1984-87*—a Review of Progress. London Health Education Authority, 1988.

NATIONAL HEART, LUNG AND BLOOD INSTITUTE. *Recommendations Regarding Public Screening for Measuring Blood Cholesterol:* Summary of a National Heart, Lung, and Blood Institute Workshop 1988.

NICHOLS, S., KOCH, E., LALLEMAND, R. J. *et al.* 'Randomised trial of compliance with screening for colorectal cancer'. *Br Med J* 1986, 293:107–10.

OLIVER, M. F. 'Problems and limitations'. In *Screening for Risk of Coronary Heart Disease.* M. OLIVER, M. ASHLEY-MILLER AND D. WOOD (eds). Chichester: John Wiley & Sons, 1987.

OLIVER, M., ASHLEY-MILLER, M. AND WOOD, D. (eds). *Screening for Risk of Coronary Heart Disease.* Chichester: John Wiley & Sons, 1987.

O'ROURKE, M. A., FEUSSNER, J. R., FEIGH, P. AND LASZLO, J. 'Age trends of lung cancer stage at diagnosis. Implications for lung cancer screening in the elderly'. *JAMA* 1987, 258:921–6.

PARKES, H. G. 'Screening for bladder cancer'. *Proc R Soc Med* 1971, 64:1267–11.

PARKES, H. G. 'Occupational bladder cancer'. *Practitioner* 1975, 214:80–86.

PUSKA, P., TUOMILEHTO, J., SALONEN, J. *et al.* 'Community Control for Cardiovascular Diseases. The North Karelia Project'. Copenhagen: World Health Organisation, 1981.

PUSKA, P., SALONEN, J. T., NISSINEN, A. *et al.* 'Changes in risk factors for coronary heart disease during 10 years of a community intervention programme'. (North Karelia Project). *Br Med J* 1983, 287:1849–4.

RASTAM, L., LUEPKER, R. V., MITTELMARK, M. B., MURRAY, D. M., SLATER, J. S. AND BLACKBURN, H. 'Population screening and referral for hypercholesterolemia.' *Am J Prev Med* 1988a, 4:249–54.

RASTAM, L, LUEPKER, R. V. AND PIRIE, P. L. 'Effects of screening and referral on follow-up and treatment of high blood cholesterol levels'. *Am J Prev Med* 1988b, 4:244–8.

ROSE, G., HAMILTON, P. J. S., COLWELL, L., AND SHIPLEY, M. J. 'A randomised controlled trial of anti-smoking advice: ten year results'. *J. Epidemiol Comm Health* 1982, 36:102–8.

ROSE, G. A. 'CHD risk factors as a basis for screening'. In *Screening for Risk of Coronary Heart Disease*. M. OLIVER, M. ASHLEY-MILLER, AND D. WOOD (eds) Chichester: John Wiley and Sons, 1987.

ROSE, G. A. 'Cardiovascular Diseases'. In *Oxford Textbook of Public Health*. Second Edition. W. W. HOLLAND, R. DETELS, AND E. G. KNOX, (eds). Volume 3. Section G. Applications and Interventions in Public Health. Oxford: Oxford University Press, 1990.

ROYAL COLLEGE OF GENERAL PRACTITIONERS' Working Party on Prevention. *Prevention of Arterial Disease in General Practice*. London: RCGP, 1981.

RUSSELL, M. A. H., WILSON, C., TAYLOR, C. *et al*. 'Effect of general practitioners' advice against smoking'. *Br Med J* 1979, 2:231–5.

SEATON, ANTHONY. 'Control of substances hazardous to health'. *Br Med J* 1989, 298:846–7.

'Secondary Prevention of Coronary Disease with Lipid-lowering Drugs'. *Lancet* 1989, i:473–6.

SECRETARIES OF STATE. *Promoting Better Health*. CM 249. London: HMSO, 1987.

SHAPER, A. G. Personal communication 1989—comment on the National Audit Office Report entitled *National Health Service: Coronary Heart Disease*.

SHAPER, A. G., POCOCK, S. J., PHILLIPS, A. N. AND WALKER, M. 'Identifying men at high risk of heart attacks: strategy for use in general practice'. *Br Med J* 1986, 293:474–9.

SHAPER, A. G., POCOCK, S. J., PHILLIPS, A. N. AND WALKER, M. 'A scoring system for identifying men at high risk of a heart attack'. *Health Trends* 1987, 19:37–9.

SHAPIRO, S. *An experiment to change detection and management of mental mobidity in primary care*. Washington, DC: National Institute of Mental Health, 1985.

SMITH, W. C. S., KENICER, M. B., MARYON-DAVIES, A. AND YARNELL, J. 'Blood cholesterol: is population screening warranted in the UK?' *Lancet* 1989, i:372–3.

SOUTH-EAST LONDON SCREENING STUDY GROUP. 'A controlled trial of multiphasic screening in middle age: results of the South-East London screening study'. *Int J Epid* 1977, 6:357–363.

TUNSTALL-PEDOE H. 'Who is for cholesterol testing?' *Br Med J* 1989, 298:1593–4.

TUNSTALL-PEDOE, H., SMITH, W. C. S. AND TAVENDALE, R. 'How-often-that-high graphs of serum cholesterol'. *Lancet* 1989, ii:540–2.

US PREVENTIVE SERVICES TASK FORCE. *Guide to Clinical Preventive Services. As Assessment of the Effectiveness of 169 Interventions.* Baltimore, Maryland: William and Wilkins, 1989.

VETERANS ADMINISTRATION COOPERATIVE STUDY GROUP. Effects of treatment on morbidity in hypertension. I. 'Results in patients with diastolic pressures averaging 115 through 129mmHg'. *JAMA*1967, 202:1028–34.

WAINE, COLIN. 'Everyone's Business—Everyone's Responsibility.' *J Roy Coll Gen Practit* 1989, 39:395–10.

WALKER, M. AND SHAPER, A. G. 'Understanding coronary heart disease: screening and prevention'. *Practice Nurse*, February 1990, 404–6.

WALLER, J. AND MORGAN, M. A. *Review and Analysis of Health Promotion and Health Education for Chronic Disease.* Report prepared for the United Health Organisation. Department of Community Medicine, United Medical and Dental Schools of Guy's and St Thomas's Hospital London, 1987.

WALLER, JANE AND MORGAN, MYFANWY. *The Use of Preventative Measures in Primary Care.* Report prepared for the World Health Organisation, 1988.

WALLER, J. AND MORGAN, M. *Prevention of arterial disease in general practice.* Report from General Practice No. 19. London: Royal College of General Practitioners, 1981.

WHO EUROPEAN COLLABORATIVE GROUP. 'European Collaboative Trial of Multifactional Prevention of Cononary Hearth Disease. Final Report of the six year results'. *Lancet* 1986, i:896–00.

WILSON, J. M. G. 'Multiple screening'. *Lancet* 1963, ii:51–4.

WINAWER, S. J. AND MILLER, D. 'Screening for Colorectal Cancer'. *Bull Who* 1987, 65:195–211.

ZUNG, W., MAGILL, M., MOORE, J. AND GEORGE, D. 'Recognition and treatment of depression in a family medicine practice'. *J Clin Psychiatr* 1983, 44:3–6.

6 SCREENING IN ADULT WOMEN

As in most cases the woman is still the
linchpin of the family, it is obviously worth
making sure that she is as healthy as
possible so that she is up to meeting the
demands made upon her.
(COOK, 1987)

INTRODUCTION

WOMEN IN GENERAL THROUGHOUT THEIR LIVES HAVE
more frequent contact with the health care services
than men, particularly at the level of primary care.
They consult not always on their own behalf but at
certain periods acting as custodians of the health of
their babies and children and the whole family. Rightly
or wrongly, it is also still to a large extent women who
take major responsibility for such matters as family
planning. The opportunities for contact with health
professionals in adult women are summarised in Table
17.

The main causes of death in women in adulthood, in
the two age-groups discussed for men in Chapter 5—

TABLE 17. *Opportunities for health service contact in adult
women*

LOCATION	TYPE OF HEALTH PROFESSIONAL
General practice	GP, health visitor, practice nurse
Hospital	Specialist medical or paramedical hospital staff as appropriate
Community	Dentist, chiropodist, family planning clinic, well-woman clinic, optometrist, pharmacist
Work	Occupational health physician, company doctor

25–44 years and 44–64 years—are shown in Table 18. The main differences between the sexes are worth noting. In the younger age group, the percentage of

TABLE 18. *Main causes of death in adult women* (England and Wales 1986)

CAUSE	NUMBER		% TOTAL DEATHS	
Young adulthood (25–44 years)				
Malignant diseases	2585		47·2	
External causes				
Motor vehicle accidents	216		3·9	
Suicide	297	950	5·4	17·3
Others	437		8.0	
Circulatory disease				
IHD	249	781	4·6	14·3
Others	532		9·7	
Diseases of the nervous system including mental disorders	308		5·6	
Respiratory disease	202		3·7	
Other causes	654		11·9	
	5480		100	
Middle age (45–64 years)				
Circulatory disease				
Ischaemic heart disease	6439		18·6	
Other heart disease	889	10721	2·6	31·0
Cerebrovascular disease	2482		7·2	
Others	911		2·6	
Malignant disease				
Trachea, bronchus, lung	2838		8·2	
Breast	4658		13·5	
Alimentary tract	2600	16665	7·5	48·2
Others	6569		19·0	
Respiratory disease (including bronchitis)	2140		6·2	
Other causes	5020		14·5	
	34546		99·9	

women dying from external causes including motor vehicle accidents and suicide is half that in men, and the percentage of those dying from circulatory and heart disease is very much lower. For nervous and mental disorders, respiratory disease and other causes, men and women are about the same. But women have double the chance of dying from malignant diseases as their male counterparts. In the 45–64 year age group, women begin to catch up in relation to death from heart disease but remain decisively in the lead in death from malignant disease.

In this chapter we will look in detail at the current screening programmes for cancer of the cervix, which illustrate many of the problems which surround the enthusiastic but unsystematic introduction of screening, and for cancer of the breast which is currently being established. We will also consider very briefly the question of screening for osteoporosis and diabetes. Screening for psychiatric diseases, particularly depression, although common to both sexes, is discussed briefly in Chapter 5.

CERVICAL CANCER

It is claimed that the vast majority of cervical cancers (theoretically up to 90 per cent) could be prevented if all women were offered and complied with high quality cytological screening programmes (Berrino 1988). A national cervical screening programme was established in the United Kingdom in 1964.

The current national policy is to screen women aged between 20 and 64 at least every five years. The 1990 contract for general practitioners (Health Departments of Great Britain 1989) contains two target levels of 50 per cent and 80 per cent of women eligible for cervical cytology in general practice. The targets will be reached and payment made if 50 per cent or 80 per cent of women aged 25–64 years in England and Wales or 20–60 years in Scotland on a GP's list 'have had an adequate cervical smear test during the previous 5·5 years'. Some of the possible difficulties involved in meeting these targets have been reviewed recently by Ross (1989).

The Strong Report on the Cervical Cytology Service in Scotland (1986) recommends screening at intervals of three years for all eligible women between the ages of 20 and 60 years. The results of a collaborative study of 10 screening programmes in eight countries to estimate the risks of cervical cancer associated with different screening policies suggested that screening should be aimed principally at women aged 35–60 years but should start some years before age 35 and that intervals between screening should be three years or less (IARC 1986). The study showed that screening every five years offered a high degree of protection but appreciably less than that given by screening every three years. There is little advantage to be gained by screening every year (Table 19). There seems to be agreement, therefore, that women eligible for cervical screening should be those in the age range 20–64, and that screening should be carried out at least every five years and preferably every three years.

However, the national programme has not yet resulted in the expected reduction in mortality from cervical cancer (Roberts 1982, Murphy, Campbell and

TABLE 19. *Percentage reduction in cumulative rate of invasive cancer in women aged 35–64 with different frequencies of screening**

SCREENING INTERVAL (YEARS)	% REDUCTION IN CUMULATIVE INCIDENCE	NO. OF TESTS
1	93·5	30
2	92·5	15
3	90·8	10
5	83·6	6
10	64·1	3

*From IARC (1986) and reproduced by kind permission of authors and publishers.

Goldblatt 1988), although as the ICRF Co-ordinating Committee on cervical screening (1984) pointed out

> with the exception of stopping the population from smoking, cervical cytology screening offers the only major proved public health measure for significantly reducing the burden of cancer today.

Various studies have shown that a reduction in mortality and morbidity is most marked in areas with comprehensive and systematic screening programmes such as British Columbia (Boyes et al 1982), Iceland (Johannesson et al 1982), Denmark (Berger 1979), Sweden (Patterson et al 1985), Finland (Hakama 1978, 1982), and some areas of Scotland (Duguid et al 1985; Macgregor et al 1985). In Norway by contrast where there has been only limited screening, there has been no demonstrable decrease in mortality (Houge 1980). And in the United Kingdom where the provision and quality of cervical cytology programmes varies widely across the country, the results of more than 20 years of cervical screening have been extremely disappointing. Within the United Kingdom, Scotland would seem to have a lower rate of mortality than England and Wales, but this is misleading. If figures for the two regions of Grampian and Tayside, where there are well-established screening programmes and more comprehensive coverage of the population, are removed, the rates for 1978 for the rest of Scotland were similar to those in England and Wales (Macgregor and Teper 1978).

The reasons for the failure of the national screening programme in the United Kingdom have been extensively examined and discussed. It is generally agreed that the problem is not so much of one of money or of expertise but of organisation, accountability, and commitment (Roberts 1982; Richards 1984). Of course it is unrealistic to expect that any non-communicable disease in adults can be completely controlled by a screening programme as Chamberlain (1984) has pointed out. There are various points at which a screening system may fail—it may fail to reach all of the target population, it may fail to be sufficiently sensitive and frequent to detect all cases, it may fail to follow up all cases detected, and treatment when instigated may fail to cure or contain the disease. The British system has been subject to most if not all of these failings.

Effective implementation of screening has various requirements which have been clearly described (ICRF Co-ordinating Committee on Cervical Screening, 1984; Intercollegiate Working Party on Cervical Cytology Screening 1987; Smith and Chamberlain 1987). In 1984, the ICRF Co-ordinating Committee on cervical screening recommended a more organised and systematic approach. They drew attention to the fact that screening had tended to be applied differentially to women at least risk of developing cervical cancer while leaving those at high risk largely unscreened, and they summarised the extensive public debate on the reasons for this as follows.

1. Most cytological examinations are performed during examinations for obstetric or contraceptive purposes leaving women in the age range of maximum risk (age 40 years and over) relatively neglected.

2. The length of the prescribed screening interval (five years) and the lack of clear and well-publicised arrangements for undergoing examination do not encourage women to attend for a smear.

Based on examination of experience in Scandinavia, the Committee suggested that a successful screening service has at least seven basic requirements and these are summarised in Table 20.

A *Lancet* editorial (1985) pointed out that most successful cervical screening programmes have three main points in common. Firstly, they are organised as public health, cancer control programmes with the specific objective of reducing mortality. Secondly, they call the age groups at greatest risk (those aged over 30 years) and they persist. They concentrate first on women who have never had a smear and they use population registers. Thirdly, there is a specific indivi-

TABLE 20. *ICRF Co-ordinating Committee (1984)
requirements for a successful cervical screening
programme**

1 Satisfactory resources for taking, examining, and reporting
   on smears
2 Acceptable arrangements for making and keeping
   appointments for examination
3 Acceptable arrangements for actual taking of smears—for
   example, choice between GP or well-woman clinic
4 Accurate listing of women in target population to enable
   complete initial call of eligible women and ensure regular
   recall as appropriate
5 An informed client population who know and understand
   the function of the procedure
6 Continuing scrutiny of records to ensure appropriate
   follow-up
7 Ability to monitor and efficiency and effectiveness of the
   programme and to adjust policies and procedures
   accordingly

*From ICRF (1984) and reproduced with kind permission of
authors and publishers.

dual in charge of screening who is responsible and
accountable for the programme. In the United Kingdom,
and in Norway, the objectives of screening were stated
in procedural terms—to provide a cytology service—
rather than in terms of outcome—to reduce mortality.
The policy of concentrating on older and never
screened women has not been implemented and it is no
one's specific responsibility to see that it is. 'The blocks
to effective action were neither scientific nor technical
but administrative' (*Lancet* 1985).

A successful screening service for cervical cancer
must depend, we would argue, on three basic and
practical elements which apply to screening in general.
Firstly, and absolutely fundamental to the success or
failure of the system, there must be an accurate,
computerised data base which is continually updated to
enable the right target population to be invited for
screening and followed up. Secondly, women must be
treated with respect as individuals who are presumed to

care about their own health. They must be given the necessary information about the smear test and its implications and offered choice of time and location when invited for screening. If the service wants to encourage women to be screened, then the onus must be on the service to make itself attractive, understandable, and accessible to the particular population involved. Thirdly, one person in each health district or health board area must be responsible and accountable for the screening programme.

These three elements are closely interrelated. The data base is essential to make sure that all eligible women are invited for screening and appropriately recalled; putting the onus on the service to sell itself to those invited is essential to ensure high compliance which should lead to the reduction in mortality that has so far eluded us; making one identifiable individual responsible and accountable for screening should be a guarantee that the system is properly established and monitored and that the follow-up and quality control implied in the invitation to be screened is satisfactory.

The data base

It could be argued with hindsight that the money spent on establishing the cervical screening programme in 1964 would have been spent more wisely on creating an accurate population index for health purposes in every health district or health board area in the country. But it is easy and usually idle to argue with hindsight. It is, however, clear that the age-sex registers of the family practitioner committees in England and Wales and the equivalent community health index in Scottish health board areas are inadequate, and it is now essential for a government committed to health promotion and disease prevention to provide adequate resources to create an accurate, updateable, computerised data base. Beginnings have been made and there are islands of excellence but the data base should exist in same form throughout the country.

As Day (1989) has recently commented

it is an astonishing aspect of this country's health service that those responsible for preventive medicine do not have an adequate list of the population giving age and sex, and equally astonishing that the lists which do exist are only for administrative purposes, for use by those with no medical responsibilities.

This problem is well illustrated in a study in an inner London district undertaken after district health authorities had been instructed to operate a cervical cytology call and recall screening programme using the age-sex registers held by family practitioner committees (Beardow, Oerton, and Victor 1989). Out of 686 invitation letters sent to women by the family practitioner committees, 477 (69 per cent) were either inaccurate or inappropriate. Overall, 90 women attended for smear. Ninety-four letters were returned by the Post Office— either the addresses were incomplete, the person concerned had moved, or the building had been demolished. A further 98 women were not eligible for a smear having recently had one, and one person invited was a man. The 404 non-responders were sent a questionnaire.

Seventy-five of these were returned undelivered and 255 received no reply—personal visits to the latter showed that 151 of the women had moved from that address. Of the 74 women who completed the questionnaire, 41 considered themselves ineligible for screening, 32 because they had had a smear within the past three years, five because they had had a hysterectomy, and four because they were virgins.

As these authors point out, their results, although possibly exacerbated in a deprived inner city area with high mobility, do have wider implications for the success or failure of both cervical cancer and other screening programmes. About half of the invitations sent did not reach the women concerned because they had moved. A further fifth of the invitations were inappropriate for various reasons. Outside the conditions of a research study where personal follow-up visits were possible, these women would have been wrongly identified as non-responders. It is also of concern that details of some smears taken within the past three years had not been appropriately recorded. The quality of the family practitioner committees age-sex registers in England and Wales or the community health index in Scotland—in theory the most accurate and extensive population indices available—is fundamental to the success of the screening programme and appears to be gravely deficient. In a study in an urban practice in London, Rang and Tod (1988) found that 30 per cent of invitations to women eligible for screening were returned as 'not known at this address', and a further 45 per cent did not reply. And even in a small stable general practice population, Ross (1989) found that between 2 and 4 per cent of patients eligible for screening could not be traced.

Bowling and Jacobson (1989) have also drawn attention to the fact that screening will fail if population registers are not improved. They cite a recent survey of the health of all people aged 85 years and over living at home in City and Hackney Health Authority which found that two-thirds of 3018 addresses on the family practitioner lists in 1986 were inaccurate (Bowling, Leaver and Hoeckle 1988). They make the valid point that between three-quarters and nine-tenths of the population consult their general practitioner during a year and consultation rates are higher among women and the elderly, both important target groups for current screening programmes and case-finding (OPCS 1986). If receptionists routinely checked patients' names and addresses when they consulted and immediately notified changes to the family practitioner committee or health board, addresses could be updated for most patients at little cost.

The women at risk

A change of emphasis from putting the onus on women to seek out the service to asking the service to attract the women is crucial to success. There is a danger in any large national programme that the concept of the individual is lost in the mass of tests to be processed and data recorded. But every woman invited for screening is an individual in her own particular circumstances with her own set of beliefs and fears about health and disease. It therefore seems logical that there is more likelihood of a woman accepting an invitation to be screened if the reasons and potential benefits of the test are properly explained and she is offered some choice in the timing and location of the appointment. Hiscock and Reece (1988) found that most of the 91 (4·8 per cent) patients in their study found to have cervical intraepithelial neoplasia would have been missed if they had not been actively encouraged to attend for screening, and in 87 of these, the abnormality was found at an early stage when treatment offers excellent results.

Standing and Mercer (1984) in a study of cervical screening in general practice achieved a smear uptake rate of 96 per cent for all eligible women—100 per cent for eligible women under 35 years of age, 94 per cent for those over 35. They acknowledge that the success of their scheme was helped by having a stable personal list of patients, most of whom were known to the general practitioner. Uptake rates are bound to vary according to turnover rate of patients and their age and social class. Local factors will also influence the best method of taking smears. In this particular practice in a compact urban setting, the nurses backed up by the general practitioner worked best for effective screening. In inner cities, family planning and well-woman clinics may be more appropriate. Standing and Mercer emphasise the need for a change in the attitudes of general practitioners to practical organisation, record keeping and preventive medicine.

In a prospective, randomised controlled trial in a group practice with a list of 10,120 patients, Pierce and colleagues (1989) examined three different approaches to screening for cervical cancer (1) a traditional screening approach with all women at risk being sent a written invitation to have a smear test; (2) a systematic opportunistic screening or case-finding approach with the notes of eligible women being tagged to remind the doctor to ask at any consultation about taking a smear; (3) an unsystematic opportunistic approach which relies on the doctor to raise the subject of a smear test during routine consultation without any reminder in the notes of eligible women. Not surprisingly, they found that systematic methods of call and recall were more effective than a non-systematic approach in encouraging women to have a smear but there was no significant difference between the two systematic methods at the end of the year of study.

It has been shown that older women dying of cervical cancer are likely not to have had a cervical smear test (Ellman and Chamberlain 1984). However, in the study just described (Pierce *et al* 1989) the response rate was not affected by age and the findings suggest that if women were invited to have a smear test by a doctor they would accept irrespective of age.

The current failure of the screening programmes to screen women at high risk seems to be due in large part, therefore, to a failure of the system to tell such women of the need for a test and invite them for screening at a convenient time and place rather than from a reluctance or refusal on the part of the women to respond positively to the invitation.

Pierce and co-workers (1989) also found that women who had had a smear test previously were more likely to respond positively to another invitation. Since more younger women are having smear tests, coverage is likely to improve in the future as women who have got used to the idea of having regular smears and who regard it as good health practice to do so, move up the age spectrum.

The question of choice of location for screening is quite important. There are those who are strongly opposed to opportunistic screening, partly on the very legitimate grounds of duplication of testing and over-load on laboratory staff. However, some flexibility is surely necessary and opportunistic screening will continue to be essential if the system is to try to achieve maximum coverage. As Cook (1987) has pointed out, unless screening is treated practically it will still be the articulate predominantly middle-class women who will benefit most.

> For women living in the middle of wasteland housing estates or in country villages with little public transport, a visit to a screening centre might mean a protracted and difficult journey, often accompanied by several small children. In the end it all becomes too much trouble.

Rang and Tod (1988), for example, emphasise that in areas with a highly mobile population, possibly at increased risk from cervical cancer, the case for opportunistic screening by the general practitioner and in gynaecological and genitourinary clinics remains strong. It is, however, essential to the success of any screening programme that results are sent to the general practitioner and information is centrally collated and recorded. They also suggest that women should be encouraged to take responsibility for their own screening—each woman screened should receive a written report with the result of her test and a date for the next smear. This seems an excellent idea, in line with the whole concept of making the service attractive and accessible to women, and similar to the system of regular appointments with optometrist and dentist.

Cervical screening seems to be most effectively based around general practice although in certain areas, such as deprived inner cities, and among certain minority groups, a different approach may be necessary. As Havelock and her colleagues (1988) point out, the general practitioner is in a good position to offer information and re-assurance about the test, especially to older women who no longer attend antenatal, postnatal, or family planning clinics and whose opportunities for screening are therefore reduced. Among other advantages of a patient being screened in primary care is the fact that the result will come direct to the general practitioner, be filed in the patient's records, and be accessible at any time (Ross 1989).

Responsibility for screening

The single factor of appointing one individual in each health district or board who is responsible for screening and accountable for the service is one that has been very much to the forefront in recent discussions on screening. Various types of health professional are involved in a cervical cytology service and co-ordination and communication can slip. The designation of one responsible person at sufficiently senior level should ensure smooth running of the system and satisfactory follow-up and quality control—all implicit in the invitation to be screened.

Preliminary results from a study of a district based call scheme in East Berkshire in 1986 showed a 25 per cent increase in uptake of screening in women with no history of screening (Havelock et al 1988) and suggest that a co-ordinated scheme with co-operation between the appropriate health authority and individual practices can improve coverage substantially.

In terms of follow-up, one of the essential conditions of any screening programme is that effective treatment is efficiently offered to all patients with abnormal results. When screening is actively proposed to asymptomatic people, the authorities encouraging the screening have a clear responsibility not only to provide such treatment but to document and monitor its effectiveness. Elwood and colleagues (1984) assessed outcome for all 1062 women who had a first report of abnormal cervical cytology in 1981. Satisfactory follow-up could be found for only 628 (59 per cent). For 275 (26 per cent) one subsequent normal smear had been reported but no other follow-up requested. For 43 (4 per cent) no subsequent test, after the abnormal smear, had been requested by the patient's general practitioner. Thirty patients (3 per cent) did not respond to a request for follow-up. Even after extensive efforts, outcome could not be established in the remaining 86 (8 per cent) of patients.

Kinlen and Spriggs (1978) looked at 101 women in Britain who had positive cervical smears, but after at least two years had escaped biopsy. Thirty-one were untraceable. Among the remaining 70 women there were 10 cases of invasive and three of micro-invasive carcinoma. The death rate in the 100 cases was 5 per cent compared with a death rate of 0·27 per cent in 4097 women in British Columbia treated for intraepithelial neoplasm grade III or more advanced lesions.

A recent report of the Intercollegiate Working Party on Cervical Cytology Screening stated that a disturbingly high proportion of women who had abnormal smears had not been investigated adequately (Sharp *et al* 1987), and Singer (1986) has suggested that many screening centres report satisfactory follow-up and management for only 60 per cent of cases. Robertson and colleagues (1988), in a follow-up study of 1347 women with mildly dyskaryotic smears for whom a repeat smear test was recommended, reported 434 (32 per cent) cases in which the woman was lost to follow-up before the implications of the abnormality could be evaluated.

One of the conclusions of an examination of a series of 173 women with cervical cancer in 1982 was that the follow-up of abnormal smears was poor because of lack of organisation, commitment, and a clear and consistent policy (Chisholm 1984).

Thus it seems clear that some women whose smears are positive are not being adequately followed up and this is an appalling finding after more than 20 years of a national programme of cervical screening. It would be the urgent responsibility of the screening supervisor to change this, and a recent report of a study in Melbourne, Australia describes a reminder system that should work in any country that provides screening for cervical cancer (Mitchell and Medley 1989). These workers studied response to the recommendation for early repeat smears in two groups of women whose initial cytological abnormalities were not considered sufficiently serious for immediate referral to a gynaecologist. If a repeat smear had not been received within three months of the recommended date a reminder letter was sent to the doctor who had taken the smear. They achieved response rates of 90 per cent and 82 per cent in the two groups and compliance increased with increasing age. As these authors point out

> Achieving high rates of follow-up smear tests and management in women with lesions that may be precursors for cervical cancer is critical to the success of a screening programme. Implementing fail-safe systems for ensuring that such abnormalities are not overlooked deserves a high priority in the design of screening programmes.

We would go further and say that, while no system can be expected to perform perfectly, a national screening programme without an excellent standard of follow-up is unethical.

Quality control is another area of great importance in a national screening programme. It is not acceptable to have widely varying standards of service in different areas of the country. As Berrino (1986) has emphasised, screening programmes should be backed by effective quality control systems as well as by the monitoring of efficacy and side-effects, health education, and standardisation of diagnostic and therapeutic protocols.

There are quality control systems in operation in this country such as, for example, one involving some 16 laboratories in Scotland where three main aspects are assessed—staining and preparation of slides, presence or not of cells, and reporting. These laboratories are now using standard forms and terminology at least for the purposes of the quality control circuit (Mann personal communication 1989).

As Smith, Elkind and Eardley (1989) have pointed out, prompt examination of smears demands considerable resources—in an average sized district about 20,000 smears a year will be examined. Truly important cytological abnormality signifies neoplastic change which is likely, without treatment, to proceed to invasion. However, the prevalence of truly important cytological abnormality is probably between 0·02 per cent and 0·3 per cent—certainly well below 1 per cent. The prevalence of reported abnormality in most screening laboratories is higher than this and thus many innocent abnormalities are being detected which we cannot distinguish from those that are significant. This has obvious and important implications both for the women concerned and for health service resources. One of the major risks associated with cervical cancer screening is probably over-treatment at various levels of severity.

Smith and colleagues (1989) also state that examining smears when well over 90 per cent are expected to be normal is very different from examining specimens from people with important symptoms and an expectation that many will be abnormal. In almost all simple screening procedures there will be a high proportion of false-negative results unless independent re-screening is built into the system. Few laboratories seem to have satisfactory internal assessment of quality, and almost none have external assessment. A serious difficulty also is that agreement among competent observers is not good. This would be a clear area of priority for a screening supervisor and the eventual aim should be national guidelines and standards of quality control.

Summary

The national screening programme for cancer of the cervix in the United Kingdom is still beset by a number of serious difficulties. The principles of a good management system for cervical screening are well understood (Hobbs *et al* 1987). It should aim to reach the entire target population and ensure recall as appropriate. The invitation to attend should explain the purpose and implications of the test and whoever is providing the service should try to deal in advance with women's anxieties. There should be some choice in regard to time and location of the test. There must also be prompt reporting of results with effective follow-up and treatment when necessary.

More than enough has been said about the deficiencies of the system thus far. It is now necessary to concentrate on getting it right and the three simple elements discussed here would go far towards this goal.

BREAST CANCER

Breast cancer is clearly an important health problem. It is the most common form of cancer among women in the United Kingdom and accounts for 20 per cent of all female cancer deaths and 4·5 per cent of total female deaths. In 1985 15,000 women in Britain died from cancer of the breast and we have the highest mortality rate from the disease in the world.

In 1987, The Government accepted the recommendations of the Forrest Report on Breast Cancer Screening and announced the establishment of a national breast cancer screening programme by 1990. The Forrest Working Group had concluded that deaths from breast cancer in women aged 50–64 years who are offered screening by mammography could be reduced by at least one-third (Forrest Working Group 1986). They recommended screening all women in the age range 50–64 years by single view mammography at intervals of three years. Women over 65 years should be able to attend for examination if they wish.

The evidence on which the Forrest recommendations were based came mainly from two large randomised clinical trials. The first of these was the Hospital Insurance Plan of New York (HIP study) which started in 1963 in 62,000 women aged 40–69 years who were randomly allocated to either a study or a control group (Shapiro 1977). Seven years after entry into the trial, cumulative breast cancer mortality in the study group was two-thirds that in the control group (Shapiro, Strax, and Venet 1977; Shapiro *et al* 1982). This difference between the two groups was maintained up to the tenth year of the trial, and for cases diagnosed in the first 10 years, up to the fourteenth year after entry. More recently the Swedish Two Counties Trial in 133,000 women aged 40–74 years has shown a similar effect over a seven-year follow-up period (Tabar *et al* 1985). Mortality in the group randomised to screening was 31 per cent lower than that in the control group. Updated results recently reported show an increasingly significant deficit in deaths from breast cancer among the 77,092 women invited to screening in comparison with the 56,000 not invited (Tabar *et al* 1989).

Additional evidence of a reduction in mortality came from the results of two case-control studies in the Netherlands. The Nijmegen project (Verbeek *et al* 1984) selected women aged 35 years and over for breast examinations by mammography every two years. The Utrecht study (Collette *et al* 1984; De Waard *et al* 1984) selected women aged 50–64 years for an initial examination by mammography and physical examination with subsequent examinations at increasing intervals of 12, 18, and 24 months. In both studies mortality from breast cancer was substantially lower in women who accepted screening than in those who did not.

The first results of the UK Trial of Early Detection of Breast Cancer were published in 1988. Between 1979 and 1981, the trial enrolled women aged 45–64 in eight locations around the country. Annual screening by clinical examination, with mammography every second year in two of the centres (Edinburgh and Guildford) and breast self-examination in the other active centres, was provided over seven years for 45,841 women; 63,636 women were offered instruction in breast self-examination and were provided with a self-referral clinic; and 127,117 women, for whom no extra services were provided, made up the control population. Over the seven years there was a reduction in the risk of dying from breast cancer in women offered screening relative to that in the control group but no difference in mortality has so far been observed between women in the self-examination group and controls. The reduction in the mammography group was 14 per cent when no allowance was made for underlying differences in breast cancer mortality between the populations but rose to 20 per cent when adjusted for differences in pre-trial mortality rates. The differences were not statistically signficant. There was no reduction in mortality during the first five years. The authors claim that these preliminary results are consistent with the hypothesis that screening can achieve a worthwhile reduction in mortality from breast cancer but stress that further years of follow-up are needed (UK Trial of Early Detection of Cancer Group 1988). This is a somewhat curious statement and the follow-up results will be of considerable interest.

In a prospective randomised trial in women aged over 45 years in Malmo, Sweden (Andersson *et al* 1988) 21,088 women were allocated to a study group and 21,195 to a control group. Women in the study group were invited to attend for mammographic screening at intervals of 18–24 months and five rounds of screening were completed. When the trial ended after almost nine years, there had been no overall fall in mortality in the study group. But among women aged over 55 years, mortality fell by one-fifth in women who were screened despite a lower rate of acceptance among the older than the younger women. Mortality also fell in the final years of the trial and just after it finished both in the whole screened group and in those aged over 55 years. The authors concluded that their data supported previous studies showing that invitation to mammographic screening may lead to reduced mortality from breast cancer, at least in women aged 55 years and over. Once again it seems difficult to regard these results as strong evidence in support of screening.

Experience with the failure of the cervical screening programme in Britain has led to a determination that the breast cancer screening programme will be properly planned, established, and evaluated. But there are problems as Acheson (1989) has pointed out. In the first place, although much is known about the aetiology of breast cancer, it is still not possible to prevent it. Secondly, available treatment is far from satisfactory in that about two-thirds of those with the disease are likely to die of it sooner or later.

The intention in the national screening programme is that for every population of half-a-million there will be a screening office as the administrative centre which will hold details of eligible women in computerised form, one or more screening units, static or mobile, and one or more assessment centres with special back-up services including ultrasonography, radiology, cytology, and histopathology. It is envisaged that the system should be organised as part of primary care in which the general practitioner with nursing support will have an essential role in inviting women for screening and giving support at every stage as necessary (Acheson 1989). The Forrest requirements for a breast cancer screening service are summarised in Table 21.

Since 1987, when the Government announced the establishment of the programme by 1990, at least one screening centre has been set up in each region and expert groups have been formed to develop guidelines on quality assurance in mammography and pathology. The UK Co-ordinating Committee on Cancer Research is developing protocols for studies to look at screening in 40–49 year olds, at the intervals between screens, and at the question of the number of mammographic views necessary. These are all important issues on which clear evidence is not yet available and research is essential.

As Frost (1988) has pointed out, incidence and mortality rates rise sharply from about age 30 years up to the age of 50 years or so and then continue to rise less steeply. No study has tried to screen women by selecting those under the age of 35 years for breast examination because the potential for saving life is small and the effect of breast examination on women under the age of 50 years is uncertain. Both in Sweden (Tabar *et al* 1985) and Nijmegen (Verbeek *et al* 1985) no

TABLE 21. *Forrest Report requirements for organisation of a breast cancer screening programme*

1	Women in the target group should be sent a personal invitation from their general practitioner
2	Arrangements for recording positive results at the basic screen must include a fail-safe mechanism to ensure that action is taken on all positive results
3	Every basic screening unit should have access to a specialist team for the assessment of screen-detected abnormalities
4	A screening record system should be developed to identify, invite and recall women eligible for screening; to record attendance for screening and results; and to monitor the screening process and its effectiveness
5	There should be adequate arrangements for quality control both within and between centres so that an acceptable standard of mammography can be maintained
6	A designated person should be responsible for managing each local screening service. The person chosen would have managerial ability and is likely to have experience in community or preventive health care, although the radiological aspects must be the responsibility of a consultant radiologist. Setting up a breast cancer screening service will require substantial managerial effort

benefit was demonstrated for women under 50 years at the start of the trial, but the number of deaths in this age group was small and the analyses are therefore subject to considerable random variation. The HIP study showed no benefit after five years of follow-up, but after 14 years the reduction in mortality seen in those who entered the trial aged 40–49 years was similar to that in those aged 50 years or more at entry. It is not yet clear whether the reduction in mortality seen in those admitted to the trial aged 40–49 is the result primarily of the examinations they received after the age of 50 years (Shapiro *et al* 1982; Day *et al* 1985; Habbema *et al* 1986; Frost 1988). Further research is needed to clarify this.

Frequency of screening examinations is also a valid topic for research. As Frost (1988) emphasises, decreasing the time between breast examinations must increase the proportion of cancers found. All current screening is done first by selecting women above a certain age and offering examination at an interval between one and three years. Tabar and co-workers (1985) suggest that pre-menopausal women should be examined every 12–18 months and post-menopausal women every 18–24 months since the mean detection lead time in the former is shorter than in the latter. The answers to questions about the interval between examinations will come from studies where those screened are randomised to different examination schedules varying perhaps from one to five years.

Forrest recommended a single-view mammographic examination and this view has been shown to have a better rate of detection than either the cranio-caudal or latero-medial views and to be a satisfactory method of breast examination (Frost 1988). However, since the cost of mammography is not greatly increased by a second view and either of the others improves the rate of detection by about 5 per cent, this also requires further evaluation.

Although the national programme is being established, the debate over screening for breast cancer continues and there are those who remain to be convinced that this is the best use of resources.

The debate can be divided into two main issues. The first concerns the practical introduction of screening in service rather than research conditions—service versus research. The second relates to the magnitude of benefit, the use of resources, and the effect on the women involved—benefit versus harm.

Service versus research

The scientific evidence on which the Forrest Working Group based its recommendations came from studies carried out in experimental trials in research conditions with highly motivated and trained staff and excellent equipment and facilities. These will be hard to replicate in normal health service practice.

Most experts agree that research evidence on the value of breast cancer screening is strong despite discrepancies when small subgroups are examined (Ellman 1987). Feig (1988) reviewed data from the five main trials of mammographic screening and reached the conclusion that annual, two view mammography with a physical examination in women aged 40 years and over could reduce mortality by at least 40 per cent and possibly by as much as 50 per cent. In routine service conditions, however, the effect on mortality is unlikely to be so high—a realistic expectation might be a reduction in mortality of between 10 and 20 per cent.

Cuckle and Wald (1988) believe that the Government has allocated sufficient funds for the national screening programme to ensure a high-quality service, provided that it is properly organised and directed. Their experience in the Reading centre suggests that this is possible and that research can be an integral part of the regular screening service. They also point out that the screening centres currently being set up are a new venture in public health for the National Health Service. They fall outside the usual structure of medical practice which is based on general practitioners and hospitals. They must be recognised as a distinct entity and allowed to function as such within the guidelines of the Department of Health.

> Perhaps most important of all, there is the need to appoint someone who would have overall responsibility for the screening service. The lack of an accountable individual with appropriate resources and authority is largely responsible for the failure of cervical cancer screening in Britain. Having learnt the lessons from that programme, Britain now has the opportunity to implement breast cancer screening effectively from the start.

High compliance is also an important factor in effective population screening (Forrest Working Party on Breast Cancer Screening 1986) and response rates of 85 per cent and more have been reported from Sweden (Tabar et al 1985) and Holland (Verbeek et al 1984). In the

United Kingdom thus far, responses have not been so favourable—60 per cent in Guildford and 61 per cent in Edinburgh (Roberts *et al* 1990).

Results of a study in which women were randomly allocated to a group receiving a letter of invitation to screening with a definite appointment time or a group which received an open-ended letter of invitation suggest that the inclusion of an appointment on the invitation significantly improves compliance with screening (Williams and Vessey 1989). This confirms earlier findings in cervical cytology screening (Wilson and Leeming 1987) and, as discussed earlier in this chapter, suggests that treating women with courtesy and encouraging them to take responsibility for their own health is sensible policy. In another study in the South-East London breast screening service, McEwen, King, and Bickler (1989) found that the overall response rate was 129 out of 283 (46 per cent) women invited but also found that 99 out of the 283 (35 per cent) did not receive their invitations. They state that the single largest contribution to increasing response rates is likely to be made by a more accurate data base and that general practitioners have an important role in counselling women whom they know have not attended for screening. This study confirms that in inner city areas with high levels of mobility, high rates of uptake will take some time to achieve.

Witcombe (1988) suggests the crucial questions are no longer whether early detection and treatment can prolong life but how far the quality of screening that has already been achieved in some research programmes can be maintained in community hospitals and what will be the cost to normal healthy women?

Training of radiologists will be essential but this will not in itself guarantee a good service. Without stringent centralised methods of quality control, screening will be demanded when skills are either not available or are inadequate. In 1987, some doubt was cast on the time scale of implementation of the Forrest Report—equipment can be bought but there are not enough radiologists and radiographers to operate the service and further training in the specialised techniques of assessment and diagnosis will be required (Ellman 1987; *Lancet* 1987). Further results from the UK Trial of Early Detection of Breast Cancer must also be awaited with interest particularly because it is the only population based study investigating whether the cheaper alternative of providing self-referral clinics for breast symptoms and teaching self-examination reduces mortality from breast cancer.

There has been extensive discussion of the value of breast self-examination in diagnosis and Hill and colleagues (1988) reviewed 12 separate published studies which related self-reported premorbid breast self-examination practices of patients with breast cancer to disease variables. They concluded that the evidence for breast self-examination as a worthwhile precaution which increases the probability of detecting breast cancer at an early stage is both more consistent and more favourable than is commonly accepted, and contend that the data they reviewed provide good grounds for encouraging women to practise breast self-examination regularly. Results of current prospective studies on this aspect in the United Kingdom (Dowle *et al* 1987) and the Soviet Union (Semiglazov and Moiseenko 1987) should help to throw further light on this.

Benefit versus harm

In 1985 Skrabanek, in an article entitled 'False Premises and False Promises of Breast Cancer Screening', contended that screening only adds years of anxiety and fear to those diagnosed and claimed that

> the philosophy of breast cancer screening is based on wishful thinking that early cancer is curable cancer, though no-one knows what is early.

In 1986 Wright examined data on screening for breast cancer and concluded that if women submitted to operation for benign disease are considered to be harmed by the screening process, then the harm to

benefit ratio could be as high as 62:1. He suggested that
mass screening for breast cancer should be abandoned
and the procedure reserved for women with high-risk
factors. Schechter and colleagues (1986) also claimed
that using a logistic model they were able to define a
high-risk subgroup and that such a selection strategy
might reduce initial visit mammography rates by up to
60 per cent with only a small reduction in case
detection. However, the results of a study by
Alexander, Roberts, and Huggins (1987) suggested that
it is not at present possible to use risk-factor information to restrict screening to a high-risk group. And, as
Alexander and co-workers (1988) further point out,
Schechter and colleagues are the only recent workers
to have been optimistic about this risk-factor approach,
their study was restricted to volunteer women in whom
50 per cent of cases have experienced symptoms, and
the complex criteria made it necessary for a woman to
attend for an examination to determine whether she
was in a high-risk category—in such circumstances, it
seems doubtful that the woman in question would
escape screening altogether although she might be
offered a simpler form of screen. Alexander *et al* (1988)
also emphasise that since it is not known whether a
policy of allocating different recall times in mass
screening would be acceptable in practice, research
would be necessary before any proposal to adopt at risk
strategy as part of public policy could be considered.

   In 1988 Skrabanek further commented that the
Forrest Report made no mention of the positive predictive value of mammography, the single most important
piece of information for any screening test. He cited the
Canadian national breast screening study, currently in
progress, where a preliminary report showed a positive
predictive value of 5–10 per cent. The implementation
of the Forrest proposals, with an estimated positive
predictive value of 5 per cent would thus result in
65,000 mammograms a year showing false-positive
results. Skrabanek goes on to point out that the harm of
screening is not confined to overdiagnosis. 'Overdiag-

nosis implies overtreatment, unnecessary biopsies, unnecessary mastectomies, and widespread anxiety and fear'.

Reidy and Hoskins (1988) state that, while we do not know what the optimal positive predictive value should be, the 33 per cent suggested by figures in the Forrest report (1986) seems too high, with the risk of missing an unacceptable number of cancers, and the 5–10 per cent quoted by Skrabanek (1988) too low, with the risk of exposing too many women to unnecessary biopsies.

The issues of fear and anxiety leading to an increase in psychiatric symptoms has also been considered. Dean and colleagues (1986, 1989) found a small percentage of women (8 per cent) who felt that breast screening had made them feel anxious about developing breast cancer. This group did have a higher psychiatric morbidity than their matched control group and it could be that a small subgroup of women are vulnerable and that screening has a detrimental effect on them from the psychological point of view. However, taking their sample as whole, these workers do not agree with the suggestion that screening for breast cancer increases psychiatric morbidity.

Ellman and colleagues (1989) support this finding. However, these authors stress that their study was carried out in a well-established screening programme in which clinical examination was included. The effect on psychological morbidity of introducing the national screening programme should be monitored. The comments of screened women indicate the importance of minimising delays in the diagnostic procedure and of maintaining full and honest communication throughout.

Warren (1988), in supporting the case for national screening, states that research results have concentrated on mortality statistics but that the benefits of screening to individual women are wider—namely, reduced morbidity and more modest surgery because of earlier diagnosis. This is a very important point and applies much more widely than simply to screening for breast cancer. In the new emphasis of screening for prevention, we must look for less crude endpoints than mortality, convenient though this is as a tool of measuring success, and we will return to this in the final chapter.

Cuckle and Wald (1988) cite three main areas of concern relevant to the issue of benefit to harm. First, there are the special ethical considerations which apply to screening apparently healthy individuals and these we have already discussed. Secondly, screening will identify only about five women out of every 1000 as having breast cancer at their first attendance and fewer at subsequent recall visits. This makes it all too easy for a screening centre to become a dehumanised production line—this must be avoided and a pleasant environment provided to encourage women to attend and to return. Thirdly, screening itself generates anxiety. Women who have abnormal mammograms and are referred for further assessment are likely to be very distressed and it is therefore vital that appropriate counselling is available and that screening should select the smallest number of women for further assessment while detecting a satisfactory proportion of breast cancers. This mean that we must accept that screening cannot detect all cases of breast cancer.

Roberts (1989) poses the question as to whether we are going the right way to provide the best possible benefit for women? Screening is always a second best, an admission of the failure of prevention or treatment, and perhaps resources currently devoted to screening would be better used for research into an effective treatment. She quotes Lippman's belief that breast cancer could be the next human cancer capable of treatment and his work on measures based on growth factors (Lippman 1988). In a paper published after her death from breast cancer in June 1989, Roberts asks what screening can actually achieve? She also challenges the 'currently expressed or strongly implied statement that if women attend for screening everything will be all right' and concludes that breast cancer screening must be brought back into its proper perspective and we must examine what it is really trying to achieve in terms of benefit for women with breast cancer.

In response, Chamberlain (1989), while agreeing that screening is not the optimal way of controlling any disease, points out that in the absence of effective prevention or treatment, it is the third best measure of control and the best available to us on current knowledge. Ellman (1989) feels that the key question concerns the means of keeping costs and emotions under control. Some choice in determining how much screening one has is reasonable and a charge for screening above what is economically justifiable from a public point of view would be the fairest and most understandable method of controlling demand. Frankness about screening is essential. Ellman concludes by stating clearly that

> the 'free' service seeks to provide a reasonable but not the maximum possible degree of protection against later development of advanced cancer and by offering further screening (with explanation of the pros and cons) to those who want to spend extra money on it we may be able to promote more realistic expectations.

We will return to this concept in the final chapter.

Summary

We would place ourselves among those who feel that there are questions that should have been asked and answered before rather than after the introduction of national screening. There seems little doubt that, under experimental conditions, screening can reduce mortality from breast cancer by around 30 per cent. We consider it most unlikely that this can be replicated under normal service conditions. And of course mortality is not the only endpoint and a great deal of damage and anguish can result from an unsatisfactory screening service. No one has yet adequately measured the disbenefits of screening, particularly in view of the number of false-positive results produced in trials so

far. Eddy (1989), in a discussion of screening in those
below 50 years of age, makes the point that it would be
worth giving the women concerned the information that
is available about the magnitude of benefit and risk and
then asking them how they feel about screening. We
must certainly move away from any idea that screening
per se is bound to be beneficial and towards the
dissemination of more complete information based on
the research findings currently available.

This particular screening bandwagon, however, is
now rolling and will be hard to stop. And, as Asbury
(1989) has pointed out, while many fear that the
programme may ultimately fail, not least because of an
inadequate data base and low compliance, we should at
least try to make it work well.

Among the most important features of the Forrest
recommendations are the insistence on monitoring of
the screening service and its effectiveness, the requirement for stringent quality control, and the designation
of one person responsible for managing each local
service. These are ingredients which, along with an
improved data base and a courteous and informed
approach to the target population, have been all too
often absent from previous screening efforts and on
them must depend the success or failure of this new
national programme.

JOINT SCREENING FOR CANCER OF
THE BREAST AND CERVIX

From time to time, it has been suggested that it might be
possible to combine screening for cancer of the breast
and cancer of the cervix on the practical grounds that it
might be more convenient for women to have both tests
at the same time and that it might also prove more cost-
effective. This has traditionally been rejected because of
the differences in age group and high-risk groups
involved in the two diseases, and at present in Britain the
different recommended intervals between screening.

However, Roberts and colleagues (1988) in a study of cervical screening at a breast screening clinic suggest that it is feasible to carry out breast screening and cervical screening at one clinic visit and that many women liked it and found it convenient. If three-yearly cervical screening were to be introduced as many people recommend, it would seem reasonable to offer combined screening to those in the 50–64 year group. As Roberts and colleagues pointed out, at least 65 per cent of women attend for breast screening when invited and the opportunity of offering a smear at the same time should not be missed. Their experience has also confirmed that women in the lower socio-economic groups are significantly less likely to attend when invited. And, as Leathar and Roberts (1985) had earlier suggested, screening might have more appeal for both older and less affluent women if it were placed in the context of total health care rather than with the emphasis placed starkly on specific disease entities.

Certainly combined screening would pose some administrative problems to begin with, but once the call-recall data base had been properly established, it should be possible, at least in the 50–64 year age group. It may be that the reasons this has not been officially considered thus far has more to do with the convenience of those offering the service than with consideration for the preference of the women involved. We would suggest further that a simple package including measurement of weight, blood pressure, questions on smoking habits, and screening for cancers of the breast and cervix in one visit should be tested for its acceptability to women.

A recent paper from Holland (Habbema et al 1990) concludes that decision-making processes in which screening programmes for breast and cervical cancer are considered separately should be abandoned. For both conditions, early detection and treatment offer the best opportunity for mortality reduction in the next decades. There are very close parallels between the two screening programmes—both aim at women only and have as their main target the prevention of disseminated cancer with its almost inevitable consequence of death. For a woman dying of cancer the untimeliness of the death rather than the site of the primary tumour is usually the predominant feature. It, therefore, seems surprising that planning and evaluation of early detection programmes for cervical and breast cancer continue to be done quite separately.

OSTEOPOROSIS

With the development of techniques such as dual photon absorptiometry and quantitative computerised tomography, it is now technically possible to measure bone mass accurately in the spine and hip (Murby and Fogelman 1987). Many centres have been established for osteoporosis screening in the United States but the value of these has been the subject of much controversy (Ott 1986; Cummings and Black 1986; Hall 1987). The US Preventive Services Task Force in its assessment of the effectiveness of 169 interventions does not recommend routine radiological screening for postmenopausal osteoporosis. Currently available procedures are time-consuming and require considerable technical expertise. The costs of screening may be justified if the burden of suffering from the disease can be reduced but further research is required to demonstrate both clinical effectiveness and cost-effectiveness. The Canadian Task Force (1988) is also against routine radiological screening for this condition.

Fogelman (1988) raises the possibility of at least one bone mass measurement for all women at the time of the menopause to assess whether they have high, average, or low bone mass. This could identify those most at risk from osteoporosis—that is, those with a low initial bone mass. He further states that improvements in technology in the near future promise higher precision measurements with very much quicker scanning times.

For the moment, we feel it would be difficult to make a

convincing case for routine screening for osteoporosis but those at risk should be offered hormone replacement therapy. This is certainly an area to be watched in terms both of current research into diagnostic techniques and of the outcome of increasing uptake of hormone replacement therapy in menopausal women.

DIABETES

Diabetes is a major health problem in the developed world. It has been estimated that the incidence of the disease is now doubling every decade, and that although dietary habits may be partly responsible for this increase, the genetic factor is the most important one.

Screening for diabetes, however, suffers from two important limitations—the lack of an accurate and practical screening test and the absence of sufficient evidence that early detection and treatment improve outcome in asymptomatic people. The main forms of treatment for mild diabetes—modification of diet and exercise—are inexpensive and of considerable health benefit to an individual generally. In Britain there is no specific policy on screening adults for diabetes.

Recommendations against screening for diabetes in non-pregnant adults have been made by the Canadian Task Force (1979) and the US Preventive Services Task Force (1989). The latter's recommendation states

> In persons who are not pregnant, primary prevention rather than screening may be an important means of preventing diabetes and its complications.

Bennett and Knowler (1984) confirm that for the majority of subjects with undiagnosed non-insulin-dependent diabetes, evidence is lacking that early detection and intervention are beneficial in preventing complications or death. They concede that these recommendations may change in the light of various research projects currently underway.

Screening for gestational diabetes is discussed in Chapter 2. And screening in certain subgroups of the diabetic population can be of benefit. As Rohan, Frost, and Wald (1989) have shown in a recent assessment, screening diabetic patients for diabetic retinopathy does satisfy the main requirements for a worthwhile screening programme. A national screening programme could prevent over 200 new cases of blindness in those under the age of 70 years each year and an estimated 60 cases in those over the age of 70.

SUMMARY AND CONCLUSIONS

Screening in adult women includes the two national screening programmes for cancer of the cervix and the breast which illustrate many of the problems surrounding the whole concept of mass screening.

Cervical cancer screening has failed thus far for largely organisational reasons. As Johnson (1989) has pointed out, in a recent review of the literature, the success of the screening programme must depend on women's motivation to take part in the screening process and their acceptance of any subsequent medical procedures. Better management and careful monitoring of the system are required and changes to the current screening programme are essential to provide a service that can meet women's needs.

In a recent statement on the Edinburgh trial of screening for breast cancer, Roberts and colleagues (1990) reported a non-significant reduction in mortality from the disease after a follow-up period of seven years; only 61 per cent of the women initially invited attended for screening. The authors conclude

> The main value of our study may be to draw attention to the manner in which defects in a programme of screening can affect mortality reduction. These defects must be recognised and remedied if the UK breast cancer screening service is to produce a significant reduction in mortality from breast cancer in women in its target

population. If these defects were to persist we would only be spending resources recklessly and to little or no effect.

With the other conditions mentioned, osteoporosis is not a candidate for screening at the moment although with increasing health awareness in the public, improvements in technology available for measurement and diagnosis, and the probable benefits of hormone replacement therapy, those at risk should be encouraged to seek advice. Diabetes, while a major health problem and by no means confined to adult women, does not satisfy the criteria for screening.

In terms of screening in adult women, therefore, we would suggest that the emphasis at present should be on ensuring that the two major current screening programmes—for cervical and breast cancer—are effectively organised, administered, and evaluated, and that there is a positive and acceptable programme of appropriate health education to encourage women to look after their health and to support them in their efforts to do so.

REFERENCES

ACHESON, D. E. *Breast Cancer Screening.* Haddow Memorial Lecture given to Section of Onocology, 28 November 1988, reprinted in *Journal of the Royal Society of Medicine*, August 1989, 82:455–7.

ALEXANDER, F. E., ROBERTS., M. M. AND HUGGINS, A. 'Risk factors for breast cancer with applications to selection for the prevalence screen'. *J Epidemiol Comm Hlth* 1987, 41:101–6.

ALEXANDER, F. E., ROBERTS, M. M., HUGGINS, A. AND MUIR, B. B. 'Use of risk factors to allocate schedules for breast cancer screening'. *J Epidemiol Comm Hlth* 1988, 42:193–9.

ANDERSSON, I., ASPEGREN, K., JANZON, L., LANDBERG, T., LINDHOLM, K., LINELL, F., LJUNGBERG, O., RANSTAM, J. AND SIGFUSSON, B. 'Mammographic screening and mortality from breast cancer: the Malmo mammographic screening trial'. *Br Med J* 1988, 297:943–8.

ASBURY, D. L. 'Breast screening: a response to Dr Maureen Roberts'. (Letter) *Br Med J* 1989, 299:1338.

BEARDOW, R., OERTON, J. AND VICTOR, C. 'Evaluation of the cervical cytology screening programme in an inner city health district'. *Br Med J* 1989, 299:98–100.

BENNETT, P. H. AND KNOWLER, W. C. 'Early detection and intervention in diabetes mellitus: is it effective?' *J Chron Dis* 1984, 37:653–66.

BERGET, A. 'Influence of population screening on morbidity and mortality of cancer of the uterine cervix in Maribo Amnt (Denmark)'. *Dan Med Bull* 1979, 26:91–100.

BERRINO, F. 'Cervical Cancer'. In *Elimination or Reduction of Diseases?* ALAN J. SILMAN AND SHANE P. A. ALLWRIGHT, (eds) Oxford: Oxford University Press, 1988.

BLAMEY, R. W. *A Cost-Effective Programme for Whole Population Breast Cancer Screening*.

BOWLING, A., LEANER, J. AND HOECKLE, T. *Survey of the needs of people aged 85+ living at home in City and Hackney*. London: Department of Community Medicine. City and Hackney Health Authority, 1988.

BOWLING, A. AND JACOBSON, B. 'Screening: the inadequacy of population registers'. *Br Med J* 1989, 298:545–6.

BOYES, D. A., MORRISON, B., KNOX, E. G., DRAPER, G. J. AND MILLER, A. B. 'A cohort study of cervical cancer screening in British Columbia'. *Clin Invest Med* 1982, 5:1–29.

CANADIAN TASK FORCE ON THE PERIODIC HEALTH EXAMINATION. The periodic health examination. *Can Med Assoc J* 1979, 121:1193–254.

CANADIAN TASK FORCE ON THE PERIODIC HEALTH EXAMINATION. The periodic health examination: 2. 1987 update. *Can Med Assoc J* 1988, 138:621–6.

CHAMBERLAIN, J. 'Failures of the cervical cytology screening programme'. *Br Med J* 1984, 289:853–84.

CHAMBERLAIN, J. 'Breast Screening: a Response to Dr Maureen Roberts'. (Letter) *Br Med J* 1989, 299:1336–7.

CHISHOLM, D. K. 'Cases of invasive cervical cancer in the North West in spite of screening'. *Br J Family Planning* 1984, 10:3–8.

COLLETTE, H. J. A., ROMBACH, DAY, N. E. AND DE WAARD, F. 'Evaluation of screening for breast cancer in a non-randomised study (the DOM Project) by means of a case-controlled study'. *Lancet* 1984,i:1224–6.

COOK, J. *Whose Health Is It Anyway?* London: New English Library, 1987.

CUCKLE, H. AND WALD, N. 'Britain's chance to get screening right'. *New Scientist* 15 October 1988, 48–51.

CUMMINGS, S. R. AND BLACK, D. 'Should perimenopausal women be screened for osteporosis?' *Ann Int Med* 1986, 104:817–23.

DEPARTMENT OF HEALTH AND SOCIAL SECURITY. *Screening for Cervical Cancer* HC84.17. London: DHSS, 1984.

DE WAARD, F., COLLETTE, H. J. A., ROMBACH, J. J., BAANDERS-VAN HALEWIJN, E. A. AND HONING, C. 'The DOM project for the early detection of breast cancer, Utrecht, The Netherlands'. *J Chron Dis* 1984, 37:1–44.

DAY, N. E., MOSS, S. *et al.* 'Screening for squamous cervical cancer: duration of low risk after negative results of cervical cytology and its implication for screening policies'. *Br Med J* 1986, 293:659–64.

DAY, N. E. 'The debate over mass mammography in Britain'. (Letter) *Br Med J* 1988, 297:1541–2.

DAY, N. E. 'Screening for cancer of the cervix'. *J Epidemiol Comm Hlth* 1989, 43:103–6.

DEAN, C., ROBERTS, M., FRENCH, K. AND ROBINSON, S. 'Psychiatric morbidity after screening for breast cancer'. *J Epidemiol Comm Hlth* 1989, 43:103–6.

DEAN, C., ROBERTS, M., FRENCH, K. AND ROBINSON, S. 'Psychiatric morbidity after screening for breast cancer'. *J Epidemiol Comm Hlth* 1986, 40:71–5.

DOWLE, C. S., MITCHELL, A., ELSTON, C. W. *et al.* 'Preliminary results of the Nottingham breast self-examination programme'. *Br J Surg* 1987, 74:217–9.

DUGUID, H. L. D., DUNCAN, I. D. AND CURRIE, J. 'Screening for cervical intraepithelial neoplasia in Dundee and Angus 1962–81 and its relation with invasive cancer'. *Lancet* 1985, ii:1053–6.

EDDY, D. 'Breast cancer screening' (Letter) *J Natl Cancer Inst* 1989, 81:234–5.

ELLMAN, R. AND CHAMBERLAIN, J. 'Improving the effectiveness of cervical screening'. *J Roy Coll Gen Practit* 1984, 34:537–42.

ELLMAN, R. Editorial: 'Breast cancer screening'. *J. Roy Soc Med* 1987, 80:665–6.

ELLMAN, R., ANGELI, N., CHRISTIANS, A., MOSS, S., CHAMBERLAIN, J. AND MAGUIRE, P. 'Psychiatric morbidity associated with screening for breast cancer'. *Br J Cancer* 1989. 60:781–4.

ELLMAN, R. 'Breast cancer; a response to Dr Maureen Roberts.' (Letter) *Br Med J* 1989, 299:1337–8.

ELWOOD, J. M., COLTON, R. E., JOHNSON, J., JONES, G. M., CURNOW, J. AND BEARER, M. W. 'Are patients with abnormal cervical smears adequately managed?' *Br Med J* 1984, 289:891–4.

FEIG, S. 'Decreased breast cancer mortality through mammography screening: results of clinical trials'. *Radiology* 1988, 167:659–65.

FOGELMAN, I. 'The case For routine bone mass measurements.' (Editorial) *Nuclear Medicine Communications* 1988, 9:541–3.

FORREST, PATRICK. *Breast Cancer Screening. Report to the Health Ministers of England, Wales, Scotland and Northern Ireland,* by a working group chaired by Professor Sir Patrick Forrest. London: HMSO, 1986.

FROST, CHRISTOPHER D. 'Breast Cancer'. In *Elimination and Reduction or Reduction of Diseases?* ALAN J. SILMAN AND SHANE P. A. ALLWRIGHT (eds) Oxford: Oxford University Press, 1988.

HABBEMA, J. D. F., VAN OORTMARSSEN, G. J., VAN PUTTEN, D. J. AND VAN DER MAAS, J. 'Age-specific reduction in breast cancer mortality by screening. Analysis of the results of the Health Insurance Plan of Greater New York study'. *J Natl Cancer Inst* 1986, 77:317–20.

HABBEMA, J. DIK F. *Combined evaluation of policies for cervical cancer and breast cancer screening.* Technical Report from the Department of Public Health and Social Medicine, Erasmus University, Rotterdam, The Netherlands, 1990.

HALL, F. M. 'Bone-mineral screening for osteoporosis'. *Am J Radiol* 1987, 149:120–2.

HAKAMA, M. 'Mass Screening for Cervical Cancer in Finland'. In *Report of a UICC International Workshop* A. B. MILLER (ed.) Toronto 1978. 93–107. (UICC Tech Rep Ser 40, 9080, 682).

HAKAMA, M. 'Trends in Incidence of Cervical Cancer in the Nordic Countries'. In *Trends in Cancer Incidence.* K. MAGNUS (ed.) Washington: Hemisphere, 1982.

HAVELOCK, C. M., WEBB, J. AND QUEENBOROUGH, J. 'Preliminary results of a district call scheme for cervical screening organised in general practice'. *Br Med J* 1988, 297:1384–6.

HILL, D., WHITE, V., JOLLEY, D. AND MAPPERSON, K. 'Self examination of the breast: is it beneficial? Meta-analysis of studies investigating breast self examination and extent of disease in patients with breast cancer'. *Br Med J* 1988, 297:271–5.

HISCOCK, E. AND REECE, G. 'Cytological screening for cervical cancer and human papillomavirus in general practice'. *Br Med J* 1988, 297:724–6.

HOBBS, P., EARDLEY, A., ELKIND, A. K., HARAN, D., PENDLETON, L. L. AND SPENCER, B. 'Synthesising research findings and practical experience to formulate principles in cervical screening'. *Cancer Detect Prev* 1987, 10:255–64.

HOUGE, N. E. 'Mass Screening for Cancer of the Uterine Cervix in the County of Ostfold, Norway'. In *Prevention and Detection of Cancer* H. E. NIEBURGS, H. E. (ed.) New York: Mariel Decker, 1980: 1875–84.

'IARC WORKING GROUP ON EVALUATION OF CERVICAL CANCER SCREENING PROGRAMMES. 'Screening for Squamous Cervical Cancer.' *Br Med J* 1986, 293:659–64.

ICRF CO-ORDINATING COMMITTEE ON CERVICAL SCREENING. 'Organisation of a Programme for Cervical Cancer Screening'. *Br Med J* 1984, 289:894–5.

INTERCOLLEGIATE WORKING PARTY ON CERVICAL CYTOLOGY SCREENING. *Report of the intercollegiate working party on cervical cytology screening.* London: Royal College of Obsteticians and Gynaecologists, 1987.

JOHANNESSON, G., GEIRSSON, G., DAY, N. AND TULINUS, H. 'Screening for cancer of the uterine cervix in Iceland 1965–1978'. *Acta Obstet Gynecol Scand* 1982, 61:199–203.

KINLEN, L. J. AND SPRIGGS, A. I. Women with positive cervical smears but witout surgical intervention. A follow-up study. *Lancet* 1978, ii:463–5.

Lancet. Editorial: 'Cancer of the cervix: death by incompetence'. *Br Med J* 1985, 2:363–364.

Lancet. 'Breast cancer screening'. (Editorial) *Lancet* 1987,i:543–4.

LEATHAR, D. S. AND ROBERTS, M. M. 'Older womens' attitudes towards breast disease, self-examination and screening facilities: implications for communication'. *Br Med J* 1985, 290:668–70.

LIPPMANN, M. E. 'Steroid hormone receptors and mechanisms of growth regulation of human breast cancer'. In *Diagnosis and Management of Breast Cancer.* M. E. LIPPMANN, A. LICHTER AND D. N. DANFORTH (eds). Philadelphia: W. B. Saunders, 1988.

MANN, EVELYN. Personal communication, 1989.

MCEWEN, J., KING, E. AND BICKLER, G. 'Attendance and non-attendance for breast screening at the South East London breast screening service'. *Br Med J* 1989, 299:104–6.

MACGREGOR, J. E. AND TEPER, S. 'Mortality from carcinoma of cervix uteri in Britain.' *Lancet* 1978, ii:774–6.

MACGREGOR, J. E. *Taking Uterine Cervical Smears.* Second Edition. Aberdeen: Aberdeen University Press, 1985.

MITCHELL, H. AND MEDLEY, G. 'Adherence to recommendations for early repeat cervical smear tests.' *Br Med J* 1989, 298:1605–7.

MURBY, B. AND FOGELMAN, I. 'Bone mineral measurements in clinical practice'. *Br J Hosp Med* 1987, 37:453–8.

MURPHY, M. F. G., CAMPBELL, M. J. AND GOLDBLATT, P. O. 'Twenty years' screening for cancer of the uterine cervix in Great Britain, 1964–1984: further evidence for its ineffectiveness'. *J Epidemiol Comm Hlth* 1988, 42:49–53.

OFFICE OF POPULATION CENSUSES AND SURVEYS. *General household survey,* 1986. London: HMSO, 1988.

OTT, S. 'Should women get screening bone mass measurements?' *Ann Int Med* 1986, 6:874–6.

PATTERSON, F., BJORKHOLM, E. AND NASLUND, I. 'Evaluation of screening for cervical cancer in Sweden. Trends in incidence and mortality 1958–1980'. *Int J Epidemiol* 1985, 14:521–27.

PIERCE, M., LUNDY, S., PALANISAMY, A. *et al.* 'Prospective randomised controlled trial of methods of call and recall for cervical cytology screening'. *Br Med J* 1989, 299:160–2.

RANG., E. H. AND TOD, E. D. M. 'Problems of cervical cancer screening programmes'. *J R Coll Gen Practit* 1988, 38:267–9.

REIDY, J. AND HOSKINS, O. Editorial: 'Controversy over mammography screening'. *Br Med J* 1988, 297:932–3.

RICHARDS, T. 'Poor organisation and lack of will have caused the failure of cervical screening'. *Br Med J* 1985, 291:1135.

ROBERTS, A. 'Cervical Cytology in England and Wales: 1965–1980'. *Health Trends* 1982, 14:41–3.

ROBERTS, M. M., LOUDON, N. B. AND HUGGINS, A. 'Cervical screening at a breast screening clinic'. *Health Bull* 1988, 46:213–6.

ROBERTS, M. M. 'Breast screening: time for a rethink?' *Br Med J* 1989, 299:1153–5.

ROBERTS, M. M., ALEXANDER, F. E., ANDERSON, T. J., CHETTY, U., DONNAN, P. T., FORREST, PATRICK, HEPBURN, W., HUGGINS, A., KIRKPATRICK, A. E., LAMB, J., MUIR, B. B. AND PRESCOTT, R. J. 'Edinburgh trial of screening for breast cancer: mortality at seven years'. *Lancet* 1990, 335:241–6.

ROBERTSON, J. H., WOODLAND, B. E., CROZIER, E. H. AND HUTCHINSON, J. *Risk of cervical cancer associated with mild dyskaryosis.*

ROHAN, T. E., FROST, C. D. AND WALD, N. J. 'Prevention of blindness by screening for diabetic retinopathy: a quantitative assessment'. *Br Med J* 1989, 299:1198–201.

ROSS, S. K. 'Cervical cytology screening and government policy'. *Br Med J* 1989, 299:101–4.

SCHECHTER, M. T., MILLER, A. B., BAINES, C. J. AND HOWE, G. R. 'Selection of women at high risk of breast cancer for initial screening'. *J Chron Dis* 1986, 39:253–60.

SEMIGLAZOV, V. F. AND MOISEENKO, V. M. 'Breast self-examination for the early detection of breast cancer: a USSR/WHO controlled trial in Leningrad'. *Bull,* WHO 1987, 65:391–6.

SHAPIRO, S., STRAX, P. AND VENET, L. 'Periodic breast cancer screening in reducing mortality from breast cancer'. *JAMA* 1971, 215:1777–85.

SHAPIRO, S. 'Evidence on screening for breast cancer from a randomised trial'. *Cancer.* June Supplement 1977, 39: 2772:2782.

SHAPIRO, S., VENET, W., STRAX, P. *et al.* 'Ten-to-fourteen-year effect of screening on breast cancer mortality'. *J Natl Cancer Inst* 1982, 69:349–55.

SHARP, F., DUNCAN, I. D., EVANS, D. M. *et al.* see *Report of the Intercollegiate Working Party on Cervical Cytology,* 1987.

SINCLAIR, R. A. AND PEDERSON, J. S. 'Screening for breast cancer'. (Letter) *Lancet* 1988, 00:1198.

SINGER, A. 'The abnormal cervical smear'. *Br Med J* 1986, 293:1551–6.

SKRABANEK, P. 'The debate over mass mammography in Britain: the case against'. *Br Med J* 1988, 297:971–2.

SKRABANEK, P. 'The debate over mass mammography in Britain'. (Letter) *Br Med J* 1988, 297:1542.

SKRABANEK, P. 'False premises and false promises of breast cancer screening'. *Lancet* 1985, 316–20.

SMITH, A. AND CHAMBERLAIN, J. P. 'Managing cervical screening'. In *Information Technology in Health Care.* Part B. Institute of Health Services Management, London: Kluwer Publishing, 1987.

SMITH, A., ELKIND, A. AND EARDLEY, A. 'Making cervical screening work'. *Br Med J* 1989, 298:1662–4.

STANDING, P. AND MERCER, S. 'Quinquennial cervical smears: every woman's right and every general practitioner's responsibility'. *Br Med J* 1984, 289:883–6.

STRONG, J. A. *et al. The Cervical Cytology Service in Scotland.* Report by Ad Hoc Group of the Histopathology Sub-Committee of the Scientific Services Advisory Group.

TABAR, L., GAD, A., HOLMBERG, L. H. *et al.* 'Reduction in mortality from breast cancer after mass screening with mammography'. *Lancet* 1985, ii:829–32.

TABAR, LASZLO, FAGERBERG, GUNNAR, DUFFY, STEPHEN, W. *et al.* 'The Swedish Two County Trial of mammographic screening for breast cancer: recent results and calculation of benefit'. *J Epidemiol Comm Hlth* 1989, 43:107–14.

'UK Trial of Early Detection of Breast Cancer. First Results on Mortality Reduction in the UK Trial of Early Detection of Breast Cancer'. *Lancet* 1988, 00:411–16.

US PREVENTATIVE SERVICES TASK FORCE. *Guide to Clinical Preventative Services.* Baltimore: Williams and Wilkins 1989.

VERBEEK, A. L. M., HOLLAND, R., STURMANS F. *et al.* 'Reduction of breast cancer mortality through mass screening with modern mammography'. *Lancet* 1984, i:1222–6.

WARREN, R. 'The debate over mass mammography in Britain: the case for'. *Br Med J* 1988, 297:969–70.

WILLIAMS, E. M. I. AND VESSEY, M. P. 'Randomised trial of two strategies offering women mobile screening for breast cancer'. *Br Med J* 1989, 299:158–9.

WILSON, A. AND LEEMING, A. 'Cervical cytology: a comparison of two call systems'. *Br Med J* 1987, 295:181–2.

WITCOMBE, J. B. 'A licence for breast cancer screening'. *Br Med J* 1988, 296:909–11.

WRIGHT, C. J. 'Breast cancer screening: a different look at the evidence!' *Surgery* 1986, 100:594–7.

7 SCREENING IN OLD AGE

No one is so old as to think he cannot live
one more year
(CICERO)

INTRODUCTION

WITH THE INCREASE IN THE PROPORTION OF ELDERLY
people in the population over the last decades, the
question of screening and preventive medicine in this
age group has attracted considerable attention. It is also
generally agreed that the health problems of the 'young'
elderly—those aged 65–74 years—should be distin-
guished from those of the elderly—those over 75 years.
In future if, as predicted, those aged 85 years and over
will almost double in numbers in the next 25 years,
there may be a case for further sub-division with a
young, middle, and old old age. What is clear is that this
is an important and increasing section of the life-cycle
as far as health care and containment or prevention of
disease is concerned.

SCREENING OR CASE-FINDING?

More than 50 years ago Anderson and Cowan (1955)
described a pioneering study in a Consultative Health
Centre in Rutherglen in Scotland set up to try to devise
methods of preventing disease in old people. This led to
considerable support for regular screening of the elderly but no consistent evidence of the benefits of this
type of approach has been forthcoming (Freer 1985).
Indeed the whole concept of multi-phasic screening has
now been discredited (South-East London Screening
Study Group 1977) and this is felt to be a poor use of
limited resources.

More recently, it has become clear that the emphasis in screening in the elderly should be on assessment of loss of function rather than on early detection of disease (Taylor and Buckley 1987). This type of intervention should try to help the elderly to lessen the problems associated with established disabilities by planned programmes of case-finding. Assessments should look at physical, mental, and social functions and, as Buckley and Williamson (1988) point out

> since the wellbeing of many older people depends on the morale and competence of informal carers the welfare needs of the carer also need to be assessed.

The importance of routine assessments, under whatever label, in this age group is based mainly upon the tendency for old people not to report disabilities which they feel they must accept as a normal part of the ageing process. There may also be an element of fear—possibly well justified in some cases—that diagnosis may result in admission to hospital or residential care.

The recent Government White Paper entitled *Promoting Better Health* (Secretaries of State for Social Services 1987) emphasised the importance of 'regular and frequent health checks for some elderly people'. Following on from this, the 1990 Contract of Service for General Practice in the National Health Service (Health Departments of Great Britain 1989) includes in its changes to terms of service in relation to health promotion and disease prevention, certain proposals relating to patients aged 75 years and over. General practitioners or other members of the practice team will be expected to offer patients in this age group the following services: a home visit at least annually to see the home environment and to find out whether carers and relatives are available; social assessment (lifestyle, relationships); mobility assessment (walking, sitting, use of aids); mental assessment; assessment of senses (hearing and vision); assessment of continence; general functional assessment; review of medication.

This approach must be generally welcomed, especially in an increasingly ageing population, although it may be rather more difficult to put into practice than the well-organised list of requirements above suggests. Many elderly people are extremely independent and may resent efforts to enquire into what they may regard as their personal affairs. However, evidence from a study of assessment and intervention in Denmark (Hendriksen, Lund and Stromgard 1984), suggested that very few of those in the intervention group who were visited every three months in their own homes felt that their personal privacy was being invaded.

It is also true that many older people are in excellent health and coping well with the inevitable rustings of age, and it does not seem sensible to insist on such a detailed assessment for everyone aged 75 years and over, regardless of perceived need. Successful application of assessment of the elderly will depend to a large extent on the skill to identify those who really require these special assessment services. As consultation data suggest that over 90 per cent of elderly patients do visit their general practitioner at least once a year, much of this assessment could be carried out in the course of a routine consultation where it might seem less intrusive —some form of mobility, for example, is suggested by the mere ability to get to the surgery. However, there is also much to be said for knowing something about the home circumstances of the elderly, and we would agree with those who suggest that an informal unscheduled annual visit would be a good use of time.

Buckley and Williamson (1988) suggest that programmes of case-finding in the elderly need two stages. The first stage involves identification of those at high risk who are likely to benefit from the second stage which is detailed assessment of function.

There are various possible ways of approaching this. One is by selecting apparently obvious high-risk groups—the very old (85+), those recently discharged from hospital, the recently bereaved, the single, and those without extended family, and so on. However, once again in this particular age group, the obvious risk groups may not be helpful in terms of need—the single and those without extended family networks, for example, may well by this stage of life have developed reliable and caring networks of friendship on which they can depend. In a study of the elderly at risk Taylor and Ford (1983) found that only the first two of these categories seemed to be valid indicators of high vulnerability. The elderly tend to be an experienced, resilient, and self-caring group.

Barber and colleagues (1980) reported the use of a postal screening questionnaire in the elderly with a full assessment of those whose answers revealed problems. Initial results produced a follow-up requirement of about 80 per cent which created difficulties with workload but the questionnaire has now been modified with a reduction in the numbers requiring follow-up.

Freer (1987) has demonstrated the feasibility of opportunistic case-finding in the elderly. He suggests that the lack of evidence to support formal screening of the elderly does not negate arguments for a 'preventive and anticipatory component to primary care' at this stage of life. A number of short screening schedules have been developed which can be used by doctors, nurses, or volunteers, or completed by the patients themselves. Patients who 'fail' the screening stage can then be fully assessed. In the pilot study in general practice, only about 28 of the 102 patients screened required follow-up and in general the doctors found the system easy to administer in normal surgery appointments.

Over 90 per cent of the over 75-year-olds see their general practitioner at least once a year (Freer 1985, Williams and Barley 1985). Consultation data also suggest that a general practitioner has on average five consultations a year with each patient aged 65–74 years and 6·3 consultations with those aged 75 years and over. Thus this type of opportunistic approach, if effectively applied, could reach the vast majority of individuals in this age group.

What we are talking about, therefore, in this last segment of the life-cycle is essentially case-finding for health and life improvement rather than screening for early detection of disease. Anderson (1976) stressed the need to look at three areas of preventive care in the elderly—physical, mental, and social—and makes the point that old people are ill not because they are old but because there is something wrong with them. We should not encourage people to expect to be ill simply because they are old.

We will now look briefly at these three areas of physical, mental, and social assessment in the elderly.

PHYSICAL ASSESSMENT

This is perhaps the area where assessment is best established and easiest to define. Many problems of physical health will have been previously diagnosed and will already be being treated. Hypertension, for example, is obviously a problem which increases with age but which is now usually diagnosed earlier in life, as discussed in Chapter 5. Clearly, the blood pressure of any elderly patient should be measured regularly during normal surgery consultation, especially in view of the fact that it now seems clear that anti-hypertensive treatment is beneficial up to the age of 80 years.

There is no scientific basis for routine assessment of the elderly for anaemia since it is a relatively uncommon problem in the general population and there is little evidence to suggest that early detection is beneficial. However, this is a clear example of where a general practitioner might make such an assessment in a patient considered to be at risk.

Hearing impairment is an increasing problem with age and is reported by 23 per cent of those aged 65–74 years, 33 per cent of those aged 75–84, and 48 per cent of those aged over 85 (US Preventive Services Task Force 1989). Elderly patients should therefore be assessed for hearing, should be given advice on the availability and use of hearing aids, and referred for further tests if necessary. At present this seems to vary from practice to practice, as does so much of assessment in this age group. However, as has already been mentioned, it is one of the specific requirements in the new contract for general practice (Health Departments of Great Britain 1989) and its application could be very beneficial. The elderly with hearing difficulties are likely to have problems in communicating with others and may suffer from increasing isolation as a result.

Problems with sight are another area of concern. Despite a general belief that such problems will have been identified and dealt with previously, a recent study (McMurdo and Baines 1988) of visual problems in geriatric patients attending a day hospital revealed a high level of severe, unsuspected, remediable, visual impairment. The US Preventive Services Task Force (1989) state the screening of vision may be appropriate in the elderly. They point out that some forms of visual impairment will lead to difficulties in walking and their correction may lessen the chance of injury and help with the functions of daily living. It is also true that many elderly people may have already had reading glasses but may need a change of prescription with increasing age. Once again assessment of vision is one of the specific services in the new contract for general practice.

With glaucoma, there is no national policy on screening in this country. Public awareness of the condition is low and many general practitioners are not aware of the difficulties it can cause but it is an important cause of blindness which can be prevented. Crick (1982) lists various risk factors for the condition including increasing age over 40 years, diabetes mellitus, family history, high level of myopia, and presence of coronary heart disease. Glaucoma is a complex condition, there is no simple universal screening test, and the only treatment is to lower intraocular pressure. There are basically three possible tests—intraocular pressure, disc evaluation and measurement, and visual field tests. None of these is satisfactory in isolation and there do not seem to be any adequate data on which combination of tests is optimal. The US Preventive Services Task Force (1989) felt that there was insufficient evidence to recommend routine screening although it may be 'clinically prudent' to recommend that those over 65 years are tested by an eye specialist.

Steinmann (1982) in encouraging optometrists and ophthalmic practitioners to be aware of their role in detecting glaucoma, suggested that screening for the condition should be part of the routine eye examination. He further stated that general practitioners should realise that the opthalmoscope may be the only tool necessary to enable them to contribute to detection provided they can recognise cupping on fundascopic examination and foster a reasonable degree of suspicion for this condition.

At present most referrals of patients with glaucoma do come through general practitioners from optometrists (Hitchings 1986). However such screening is patchy because optometrists tend to see two select population groups—those with symptoms from presbyopia in their 40s and 50s and thus below the peak age for the onset of glaucoma and those with visual symptoms of eye disease which, if caused by glaucoma, will reflect an advanced stage of the disease. Hitchings considers that general practitioners are well placed to identify asymptomatic patients with glaucoma since they see most of the elderly patients on their lists regularly, especially those with risk factors of family history, systemic hypertension and diabetes. There is, however, need for education in recognition of the condition if ophthalmic outpatient departments are not to be overloaded with query glaucomas, as is tending to happen at the moment.

Diabetic retinopathy is another important problem. As mentioned in Chapter 6, Rohan, Frost, and Wald (1989) suggest that a screening programme in diabetics under the age of 70 years will prevent an estimated 215 cases of blindness and will also prevent around 60 cases of blindness in the over 70s.

It seems clear that attention to general and specific

problems of vision in the elderly is likely to be worthwhile. Recent surveys suggest that the abolition of free sight tests in April 1989 has led to a fall in the number of tests carried out. We would suggest that those over 65 years of age should be added to the list of those exempt from payment to encourage regular testing in this particularly vulnerable group.

MENTAL ASSESSMENT

The main problems in this area for the elderly are dementia and depression. Dementia is responsible for an enormous burden of suffering but an effective screening test for its early detection remains elusive. It is also true that it does not meet the criteria for screening in that there is no cure available. Clinicians fail to detect between 21 and 72 per cent of patients with dementia, especially when the disease is early in its course, and conversely many without the disease are incorrectly diagnosed as having it (Roca *et al* 1984; WHO 1986). There is also the potential confusion of depression posing as dementia. The US Preventive Services Task Force Report (1989) does not recommend routine screening tests for dementia for elderly people with no evidence of cognitive impairment and there are no official recommendations on screening from elsewhere. There is to date no scientific evidence to suggest that dementia patients diagnosed early are less likely to experience secondary medical and psychiatric complications. However common sense and humanity suggest that early diagnosis will permit carers to work out how best to deal with the problem and seek appropriate support before it becomes too acute. The greatest benefit of early diagnosis occurs among the 10–20 per cent of dementias that are potentially reversible, such as those caused by drug toxicity, metabolic disorders, hypothyroidism, and depression (Caine 1981; Beck *et al* 1982; US Preventive Services Task 1989). Early diagnosis must therefore be welcomed. There is also a paramount need to provide support for the carers of the elderly, especially where dementia is involved, to enable them to continue to cope (Caird, personal communication 1989). This aspect of care of the elderly is vital and has been covered in some detail in the report *The Nation's Health: A Strategy for the 1990s* (Smith and Jacobson 1988).

Depression is another potential health problem in this age group and one that is probably much underestimated. As in other age groups, however, there is no satisfactory screening test or easy solution. More research is certainly needed in this area. As D'Souza (1988) has pointed out, there is also need to acknowledge the possibility that the elderly may want to feel able to discuss the prospect of death in order to prevent anxieties of pain and isolation in the process of dying. This, we would contend, has now become a legitimate part of health education—by prolonging life and making dying by and large a later and more gradual process, we must be prepared to discuss its inevitability and preparation for it. However, the increasing trend towards dying in hospital has left many general practitioners inexperienced and unsure as to how best to support the dying and their relatives at home (Haines and Booroff 1986).

SOCIAL ASSESSMENT

In this sphere of assessment, which is likely to devolve more on the health visitor and other members of the practice team than on the general practitioner, the emphasis must be on function both in a physical and social sense. However it is also here that perhaps the most apparently minor problems can make the greatest difference. The checking of feet, for example, and referral to a chiropodist if necessary, can make an enormous difference to mobility and comfort. And it is important for the general practitioner to know the home circumstances and family and social relationships of an elderly patient. These are relevant to determining the need for home visits, medical care, home helps, and the development of networks of social support, including meals on wheels, day care centres and so on, and outside contact to alleviate loneliness and improve the quality of life in those at risk from isolation.

Hendriksen and colleagues (1984) carried out a randomised controlled trial of the consequences of assessment and intervention among elderly people in a suburb of Copenhagen. Over a period of three years, 285 randomly selected subjects aged 75 years or over were visited at home every three months to assess whether medical and social intervention of this nature would influence the number of admissions to hospital or nursing home, the number of contacts with the general practitioner, or mortality. A randomly selected control group of 287 subjects of the same age and sex were visited during the final three months of the study.

There was a significant reduction in the number of admissions to hospital in the intervention group and there were 56 deaths in the intervention and 75 in the control group (p>0·05). There was no difference between the groups in the number of contacts with the general practitioner but significantly fewer emergency medical calls were registered in the intervention group. Subjects in the intervention group benefited from the regular visits and the increased availability and distribution of aids and modifications to their homes to which these led. The visits also seemed to produce an important increase in confidence through regular contact with the same person whom they could telephone to discuss particular problems.

> Even among very old people we were able to achieve an effect through preventive effort. This has wide implications in regard to future medical and social planning for the elderly ... Preventive visiting is a feasible way for the community to meet the demands of elderly people who want to stay in their own homes as long as possible. For this method to work one person must co-ordinate the

multi-disciplinary activities, be available every day, have a thorough knowledge of social and medical systems, and have an understanding and a devoted interest in elderly people.

In an earlier trial of geriatric screening and surveillance in a practice population of 295 patients aged 70 years and over, many previously unidentified medical and social problems were found. Of the medical conditions found, 67 per cent were manageable, half being improved and the remainder resolved completely (Tulloch and Moore 1979). The screening programme did increase usage of health and social services but also decreased expected duration of stay in hospital.

Tulloch and Moore (1979) suggest that effective medical care of the elderly requires a basic screening programme to identify social, economic, functional, and medical problems likely to affect their health and quality of life.

> The real pathology of old age is pain, disablement, frustration, boredom, lack of purpose, and loss of identity and self-respect, all of which lead to dissatisfaction with the quality of life.

SUMMARY AND CONCLUSIONS

In old age, more than perhaps any other segment of the life-cycle, there currently exists the potential to improve quality of life in both health and social terms by screening or case-finding in a relatively simple and inexpensive way. The simple formula of you are old therefore you die, no longer holds good. We all still have to die at some point, but we are taking a great deal longer on average to do so. The task now is ensure that quality of life is as good as it can be for the extra life years.

However, there is still an unacceptably large gap between the problems that exist in this age group and those that we identify and treat or help. Williamson (1981) in a discussion of the theoretical benefits of case-finding, showed that about 30 per cent of the problems described by the elderly when visited were unknown to health or social service personnel. There is also a pattern about the undiscovered problems (Vetter, Jones and Victor 1983). Respiratory, cardiac, and nervous system problems tend to have been previously diagnosed. Urinary problems (especially incontinence), and locomotor and mental problems (especially dementia and depression) and problems with the feet are largely undiagnosed. Furthermore social difficulties, for example with housing or carers, are less well known than physical problems.

As Vetter (1988) has recently pointed out, there is a need for more research into effective methods of casefinding in the elderly with clear measurements of its value. It is also necessary to convince the target age group that their health and wellbeing is as much the concern of the National Health Service as that of any other age group and combat the tendency of the elderly merely to accept certain remediable disabilities as the inevitable consequence of age.

The health professionals the elderly encounter must share this outlook and not dismiss legitimate and possibly serious worries about health and social circumstances too lightly. Ten years ago it was suggested that general practitioners did not see themselves as responsible for the social needs of their patients (BMJ 1979). And in a questionnaire study of disablement and care (Patrick, Peach and Gregg 1982), many disabled respondents gave prescribing as their doctor's most important role. There is no doubt that this is changing but further research and evaluation on appropriate methods of delivery of health care and social and functional support in this age group are clearly extremely important. It is also vital, as Waller and Morgan (1988) have stressed, that with the introduction of the new contract for general practice and the requirement of regular health assessments for the elderly, national guidelines are properly developed, publicised, implemented, and evaluated.

REFERENCES

ANDERSON, W. F. 'Preventive Medicine in the Elderly'. In *Social and Medical Problems of the Elderly*. KENNETH HAZELL (ed.) Fourth edition. London: Hutchison, 1976.

ANDERSON, W. F. AND COWAN, N. R. 'A consultative health centre for older people'. *Lancet* 1955, 2:239–40.

BARBER, J. H., WALLIS, J. B., McKEATING E. 'A postal screening questionnaire in preventive geriatric care'. *J Roy Coll Gen Practit* 1980, 30:49–51.

BECK, J. C., BENSON, D. F., SCHEIBEL, A. B. *et al.* 'Dementia in the elderly: the silent epidemic'. *Ann Intern Med* 1982, 97:231–41.

BRITISH MEDICAL JOURNAL. 'Are they being served?' (Editorial) *Br Med J* 1979, 1:147–8.

BUCKLEY, E. G. AND WILLIAMSON, J. 'What sort of "health checks" for older people?' *Br Med J* 1988, 296:1144–5.

CAINE, E. D. 'Pseudodementia'. *Arch Gen Psychiatry*, 1981, 38:1359–64.

CAIRD, F. I. Personal communication, 1989.

CRICK, R. P. 'Early detection of glaucoma'. *Br Med J* 1982, 285:1063–4.

D'SOUZA, MICHAEL. 'Can I prevent disease and disability?' In *Epidemiology in General Practice*. D. MORRELL (ed.) Oxford: Oxford Medical Press, 1988.

FREER, C. B. 'Consultation-based screening of the elderly in general practice: a pilot study'. *J R Coll Gen Practit* 1987, 37:455–6.

FREER, C. B. 'Geriatric screening: a reappraisal of preventive strategies in the care of the elderly'. *J Roy Coll Gen Practit* 1985, 35:288–90.

HAINES, A. AND BOOROFF, A. 'Terminal care at home: perspective from general practice'. *Br Med J* 1986, 292:1051–3.

HEALTH DEPARTMENTS OF GREAT BRITAIN. *General Practice in the National Health Service. The 1990 Contract.* August 1989.

HENDRIKSEN C., LUND, E. AND STROMGARD, E. 'Consequences of assessment and intervention among elderly people: a three year randomised controlled trial'. *Br Med J* 1984, 289:1522–4.

HITCHINGS, R. A. 'Screening for glaucoma.' *Br Med J* 1986, 292:505–6.

McMURDO, M. E. T. AND BAINES, P. S. 'The detection of visual disability in the elderly'. *Health Bull* 1988, 46:327–9.

PATRICK, D. L., PEACH, H. AND GREGG, I. 'Disablement and care: a comparison of patient views and general practitioner knowledge. *J R Coll Gen Practit* 1982, 32:429–34.

ROCA, R. P., KLEIN, L. E., ROBY, S. M. *et al.* 'Recognition of dementia among medical patients'. *Arch Intern Med* 1984, 144:73–5.

ROHAN, T. E., FROST, C. D. AND WALD, N. J. 'Prevention of blindness by screening for diabetic retinopathy, a quantitative assessment'. *Br Med J* 1989, 299:1198–201.

SECRETARIES OF STATE FOR SOCIAL SERVICES. *Promoting Better Health*. White Paper. CM. London: HMSO, 1987.

SMITH, A. AND JACOBSON, B. (eds) *The Nation's Health. A Strategy for the 1990s*. A report from an Independent Multidisciplinary Committee chaired by Professor ALWYN SMITH. London: King Edward's Hospital Fund for London, 1988.

SOUTH-EAST LONDON SCREENING STUDY GROUP. 'A controlled trial of multiphasic screening in middle age'. *Int J Epidemiol* 1977, 6:357–63.

STEINMANN, W. C., 'The "who" and "how" of detecting glaucoma'. *Br Med J* 1982, 285:1091–3.

TAYLOR, R. C. AND FORD G. G. 'The elderly at risk. A critical examination of commonly identified risk groups'. *J Roy Coll Gen Practit* 1983, 33:699–700.

TAYLOR, R. C. AND BUCKLEY, E. G. (Eds) *Preventive Care of the Elderly: a review of current developments*. Occasional Paper No. 35. London: Royal College of General Practitioners, 1987.

TULLOCH, A. J. AND MOORE, V. 'A randomised controlled trial of geriatric screening and surveillance in general practice'. *J Roy Coll Gen Practit* 1979, 29:730–3.

US PREVENTIVE SERVICES TASK FORCE. *Guide to Clinical Preventive Services*. Baltimore: Williams and Wilkins, 1989.

VETTER, N. 'Routine assessments of the elderly'. (Editorial) Update 1988 (15 October), 659–61.

VETTER, N. J., JONES, D. A. AND VICTOR, C. R. 'Effect of health visitors working with elderly patients in general practice: a randomised controlled trial'. *Br Med J* 1984, 288:369–372.

WALLER, J. AND MORGAN, M. *The Use of Preventive Measures in Primary Care*. Report for the World Health Organisation. London: Department of Community Medicine, St Thomas' Campus, 198.

WILLIAMS, E. S. AND BARLEY, N. H. 'Old people not known to the general practitioner: low risk group'. *Br Med J* 1985, 291:251–4.

WILLIAMSON, J. 'Screening, surveillance and case-finding'. In *Health Care of the Elderly*. T. ARIE (ed.). London: Croom Helm, 1981.

WORLD HEALTH ORGANISATION. *Dementia in later life: research and action*. Report of a WHO scientific group on senile dementia. Tech Rep Series 730. Geneva: WHO, 1986.

SCREENING IN BRITAIN: PRESENT AND FUTURE

8

A wise man ought to realise that health is
his most valuable possession
(HIPPOCRATES: *A Regimen for Health*)

WE HAVE TRIED IN THE PRECEDING CHAPTERS TO LOOK
at the current status of screening in Britain at every
stage of life and Table 22 contains a summary of the
present position together with our recommendations
which we discuss later in the chapter.

THE PRESENT

In the antenatal period, women attending for antenatal
care are screened routinely for syphilis and rubella at
their first visit. With Down syndrome, women aged
over 35 years and those with a previous or family
history of chromosomal abnormality are offered diagnostic amniocentesis. There is no uniformity on screening for the haemoglobinopathies or neural tube defects
and local arrangements vary. With hepatitis B virus,
HIV virus, and gestational diabetes there is no general
policy on screening although effective screening tests
are available; in asymptomatic bacteriuria there is again
no official policy in this country.

In the neonatal period, screening is carried out
routinely for phenylketonuria and congenital hypothyroidism. There is no uniform policy on screening for
other inborn errors of metabolism or for cystic fibrosis
and screening availability varies in different parts of the
country. Screening for congenital dislocation of the hip,

developmental disorders, impairments of sight and hearing, heart disease, asthma, and undescended testes are routine clinical practice but there is current discussion as to whether the tests are adequate or worthwhile.

In childhood, routine examinations of immunisation status and impairments of sight and hearing are carried out in primary care and in the education service. The new contract of service for general practice in the National Health Service (Health Departments of Great Britain 1989), with its emphasis on health promotion and disease prevention, lays particular stress on the value of immunisation with coverage targets for general practitioners. Mental and physical development are routinely assessed but there is considerable doubt about the value of this as discussed fully in Chapter 3. There is no official policy on screening for iron deficiency anaemia and once again the position varies according to locality.

In adolescence, there is routine examination of girls for scoliosis but there is doubt about the value of this and concern has been expressed about the possibility of over-treatment. There is no general policy on screening for individuals at risk of contracting rubella although national guidelines suggest immunising adolescent girls. In early adulthood there are no recommended routine screening investigations.

In adult men there is no official policy at the moment on screening for risk of coronary heart disease nor for the major cancer causes of death, nor for psychiatric disorders or diabetes. In adult women there are national screening programmes for cancers of the cervix and breast but again no official policy on screening for risk of coronary heart disease, osteoporosis, diabetes, or psychiatric disorders.

In old age, there is no general policy on screening and the position also varies across the country. However, once again the 1990 contract for general practice (Health Departments of Great Britain 1989) stresses the importance of care and assessment in the elderly, especially in those aged over 75 years. And, as we have discussed in Chapter 7, this is a stage of life when simple routine screening in general practice may uncover minor health problems which can be dealt with relatively easily and economically and make a major improvement in the quality of life and in mobility for the individual concerned.

Thus, with the exception of certain well-established screening procedures in the antenatal and neonatal periods, routine clinical examinations—some of which are of doubtful value—in childhood, scoliosis in adolescent girls, and cancer of the cervix and breast in adult women, there is no official policy on screening in this country at the present time.

We would not regard this as a negative aspect. As we have stressed throughout this book, screening should only be contemplated if certain criteria are fulfilled. A more cautious approach to proposals for screening may protect us from some of the over-enthusiasm for the practice that has been seen in some programmes in the United States where a vast amount of screening is carried out without clear benefit. An extreme example of the consequences of unrestrained screening currently reported from the United States is the demand for prophylactic mastectomy by women considering themselves at high risk from breast cancer (Helzlsouer 1990). This aspect must be emphasised particularly today in view of the change from need-led to demand-led health care, a very important change in philosophy and one that has not yet been sufficiently acknowledged.

However, there are a number of problems that arise from the lack of a general policy on basic health screening. Firstly, there are wide differences in access to screening facilities and availability of treatment for different conditions in different parts of the country and indeed between different hospitals and general practices within the same area. While it is always going to be impossible to achieve a uniform standard of health care and competence, availability of screening for a particular condition should not depend on where a patient happens to live.

Secondly, there appears to be a serious lack of co-ordination. In many areas there is no one responsible for screening activities and it is therefore easy for proper follow-up to fail. Various different types of health professional may be involved with one case or screening programme but no one takes overall responsibility and there may also be inadequate communication between them. One of the recommendations of the Hall Report (1989) is that one person within an authority should take responsibility for co-ordination of screening activities and we would endorse this whole-heartedly. The lack of any central screening responsibility is highlighted by the situation in screening for risk of coronary heart disease. As Shaper (1989) has pointed out, there is a danger that in shifting the emphasis in this type of screening to primary care, the responsibility for this major cause of death and illness will also be shifted from national to local level and its efficiency will depend on individual practices and practitioners.

Thirdly, there is very little in the way of systematic scientific evaluation of existing screening programmes without which it is impossible to judge the value of a particular programme. Evaluation is absolutely essential and should be built in to the foundations of any screening activity.

Fourthly, there is a lack of proper quality control in many screening programmes. There are quality control circuits, for example, in the field of cervical cancer screening but there is no compulsion on any laboratory to participate. In this context also we should not overlook the large number of screening tests carried out in private clinics and hospitals where evaluation and quality control may be lacking and where communication of results to the main National Health Service system may be deficient.

Finally, there appears to be a paucity of quality health education and promotion linked to screening. This must be of concern at a time of increasing public awareness of health as a positive factor and an overlap between changing lifestyles and national policies of prevention. There are encouraging signs in this area, such as the recent publication in England of a strategic plan for health education for the next five years (HEA 1989).

Conclusion

The state of screening in Britain today can fairly be described as patchy and disorganised. In some areas for some conditions, facilities are excellent but there is a lack of uniformity, an unacceptable level of variation across the country, and a dearth of systematic evaluation. And as the Hall Committee pointed out, some screening is routinely carried out in the absence of evidence of its value. What we need is not necessarily more screening. Rather we need a critical re-appraisal of current practices and agreement on a basic system of opportunistic screening and prevention according to age at primary care level nationwide with rather less emphasis on mortality as the sole endpoint than has been the case in the past. The resource implications for general practice must also be evaluated, both in terms of finance and manpower. There is a clear need to identify what is feasible within the context of screening in health care and make sure that screening programmes are properly assessed, introduced, monitored, and evaluated.

THE FUTURE

In spite of the problems summarised above, we believe that we do have the foundation for a first class screening and prevention programme, building on past experience and using our excellent primary care system.

In the past, as we have seen, screening in Britain as elsewhere has been organised very much on a disease-specific basis and the present situation with wide variations in provision and standards of screening between areas reflects this approach. There is much to be said for a more unified system as we have tried to suggest—screening for the whole individual considered by stage of life and particular risk factors rather than by disease. More and more general practices in the United Kingdom are now working from sizeable purpose-built premises and advantage of this could be taken for screening. The risk factor approach is emphasised in the United States where screening is often described as predictive medicine. We can learn a great deal both positive and negative from experience there where the concepts of screening and of health promotion have been embraced with more enthusiasm than the more sceptical and cautious British attitudes seem to allow. ˙

The emphasis in the United States, however, is now changing as illustrated in the report of the US Preventive Services Task Force *Guide to Clinical Preventive Services* (1989). The Task Force assessed the effectiveness of 169 screening interventions and recommended periodic health examinations determined by the patient's age, sex, and other risk factors in preference to the annual complete physical examination in which all patients receive the same routine battery of tests and procedures regardless of risk.

It is clear that a modern concept of screening is inextricably linked to disease prevention and health promotion, that there must be greater emphasis on case-finding and risk-factor screening, and that such activities should be based primarily in general practice. We suggest that there should be a core programme of screening tests to be carried out routinely at the different stages of the life-cycle with other specialist tests carried out only in groups of the population considered to be at risk. These recommendations are summarised in Table 22 and we will discuss them briefly here.

There are opportunities, described recently by D'Souza (1988), for pre-conception counselling and there is a growing body of opinion that routine advice should be offered to all couples intending to start a family rather than simply to those who seek genetic

TABLE 22. *Summary of current and recommended status of screening in the United Kingdom according to life-cycle stage*

LIFE-CYCLE STAGE	CONDITION	CURRENT STATUS	OUR RECOMMENDATION
ANTE-NATAL	Down syndrome	Selection of women for diagnostic amniocentesis on basis of advanced age (>35 yrs) or family history of chromosomal abnormality	Screening using amniocentesis on the basis of maternal age in conjuction with three biochemical markers and possibly also ultrasound
	Haemoglobin-opathies	No national policy—local fetal screening for at-risk groups either on request or in research context	Serological screening and chorionic villi sampling for appropriate ethnic minority groups
	Neural tube defects	No national policy—ad hoc screening arrangements satisfactory in some areas, less so in others	Routine AFP screening in high-risk areas
	Syphilis	Serological screening performed routinely at first antenatal visit	As at present
	Rubella	As for syphilis	As at present
	Hepatitis B virus (HBV)	Effective tests available	Not recommended at present. Further research needed
	HIV virus (AIDS)	No national policy Effective tests available	Not recommended at present. Further research needed

TABLE 22.—continued

LIFE-CYCLE STAGE	CONDITION	CURRENT STATUS	OUR RECOMMENDATION
ANTE-NATAL—continued	Gestational diabetes	Effective tests available	Not recommended at present. Further research needed
	Asymptomatic bacteriuria	No national policy. Doubt as to whether treatment is effective	Routine assessment in the first three months of pregnancy. Effective treatment available.
NEO-NATAL	Phenylketonuria (PKU)	Routine in the neonatal period	Routine screening as at present
	Congenital hypothyroidism (CH)	National screening established in 1982 working with the programme for PKU	Routine screening as at present in conjunction with that for PKU
	Other inborn errors of metabolism	No national policy—screening availability variable according to locality	Other conditions where early detection could be useful include galactosaemia, maple syrup urine disease, homocystinuria . . . Further research is needed.
	Cystic fibrosis	No national policy—screening availability variable according to locality	Screening may be appropriate in affected families. Better tests will soon be available using DNA technology

Congenital dislocation of the hip (CDH)	Routine clinical practice in neonatal period but doubt about whether tests are adequate or meaningful	Further evaluation of benefit essential although serious defects are likely to be identified by routine neonatal examination
Developmental disorders		
Impairments of vision/hearing		
Heart disease		
Asthma		
Undescended testes		
CHILDHOOD Immunisation status	90–100% uptake is aim	Routine examinations in primary care and education service—every opportunity should be taken to encourage uptake of appropriate immunisations to reach target
Visual/hearing impairment	Routine examinations in primary care and education service	Routine check of visual acuity and hearing in conjunction with observations from parents, teachers etc

TABLE 22.—*continued*

LIFE-CYCLE STAGE	CONDITION	CURRENT STATUS	OUR RECOMMENDATION
CHILD-HOOD *continued*	Iron deficiency anaemia	No national policy—ad hoc local arrangements and research programmes	Screening may be useful in certain ethnic minority or socially deprived groups. We do not consider that screening should be done routinely
	Mental and physical development	Routine examinations in primary care and education service but value uncertain	Changes in developmental screening practices may be evaluated first in one or two areas. No evidence that routine measurement of height or weight is beneficial
ADOLES-CENCE	Scoliosis	Routine examination with visual inspection the suggested procedure	Routine screening not recommended until there is further evaluation
	Rubella	No national policy	Efforts should be devoted to improving awareness of the potential dangers of the virus in pregnancy and providing immunisation as necessary

YOUNG ADULT-HOOD	Hepatitis B HIV Venereal disease Cigarette smoking Alcohol or drug abuse		No routine screening recommended. Every opportunity for health education should be taken
	Family planning/genetic counselling	No national policy—variable local arrangements	Referral to specialist service for those considered to be at risk
	Psychiatric disorders	No national policy—variable local arrangements	An important problem but no satisfactory screening test or solution. Further research needed
		No national policy	
ADULT-HOOD MEN	Risk of coronary heart disease Hypertension Cigarette smoking Blood cholesterol level	No national policy—emphasis on advice in primary care and health education Individual local arrangements and research projects	Screening for risk factors during normal consultation—weight, family history, cigarette smoking, blood pressure routinely; cholesterol if indicated

TABLE 22.—*continued*

LIFE-CYCLE STAGE	CONDITION	CURRENT STATUS	OUR RECOMMENDATION
ADULT-HOOD MEN *continued*	Cancer	No national policy	
	Colorectal	No national policy	Screening not recommended at present results of current research may change this
	Lung	No national policy	Routine questions about smoking habits during normal consultation
	Bladder	Takes place as part of occupational screening	Worksite screening
	Psychiatric disorders	No national policy.	An important problem but, as noted above, no satisfactory screening test or solution. Further research needed
	Diabetes	No national policy.	Not recommended routinely—further evaluation necessary
WOMEN	Cancer		
	Cervix	National screening programme established in 1964	Continuation and improvement of national screening programme established in 1964
	Breast	National screening programme established in 1988 for women aged 50–64 years	Effective establishment and evaluation of national screening programme

Risk of coronary heart disease	No national policy—emphasis on advice in primary care and health education	Screening for risk factors during normal consultation—weight, family history, cigarette smoking, blood pressure routinely; cholesterol if indicated
Osteoporosis	No national policy	Not recommended at present but those at risk should be offered hormone replacement therapy
Diabetes	No national policy	As for men
Psychiatric disorders, in particular depression	No national policy—ad hoc local arrangements	An important problem but no satisfactory screening test or solution. Further research needed. More attention to be paid to basic psychiatric training for GPs
OLD AGE		
General functions	No national policy—ad hoc local arrangements	Screening to be undertaken during normal routine consultations with referral to specialist services as appropriate.
Sight, hearing, mobility		
Psychiatric disorders: dementia, depression		Attention to be paid to those felt to be at risk of certain conditions—eg glaucoma. Eye tests should be exempt from charge.
Anaemia		
Hypertension		

counselling or are known to be at particular risk. Such advice would be centred on general practice and would include three main areas—the importance of planning a family so that children are spaced and conceived at a time when the family can best cope, a warning of the possible damage to the embryo of alcohol consumption and cigarette smoking, and the importance of adequate diet and nutrition in early pregnancy.

At the antenatal stage, core screening tests should include screening for Down syndrome, currently using diagnostic amniocentesis on the basis of maternal age. As indicated in Chapter 2, it seems likely that further work on the evaluation of examining the three biochemical markers described, with ultrasound if indicated, may modify the screening method of choice in the near future. The evidence on screening for neural tube defects is not conclusive but since AFP screening of maternal serum could be done on the sample of blood withdrawn for other purposes, we would suggest that it could be done routinely, again with ultrasound if indicated. Routine serological screening for syphilis and rubella should continue at the first antenatal visit with assessment of urine for bacteriuria at some point during the first three months of pregnancy. At-risk groups, such as appropriate ethnic minorities, should be offered serological screening and chorionic villi sampling for the haemoglobinopathies, with appropriate follow-up support and treatment. At this stage of the life-cycle, there may be some confusion about where screening takes place—in an antenatal clinic or in general practice. Wherever it is carried out, it is essential that good links are established between clinics to avoid duplication or neglect of tests and to ensure accurate recording of results and appropriate counselling.

In the immediate neonatal period, most screening will take place in hospital. The core programme here should include routine screening for phenylketonuria, congenital hypothyroidism, and severe impairments of sight and hearing as at present. Infants considered at risk because of family history, for example, should be screened for other inborn errors of metabolism, and screening for cystic fibrosis may soon be appropriate in previously affected families with improved tests currently being developed. Other serious abnormalities of, for example, the heart or obvious CDH, will almost certainly be identified in normal neonatal examination.

Routine opportunistic screening of babies and infants in the first year of life should provide sufficient supervision at this stage, within the normal framework of general practice in conjunction with the assessment of parents.

In childhood most core screening will take place at primary care level and as D'Souza (1988) has pointed out, because young children present with large numbers of viral infections at this time, most in this age group will be seen by their family doctor. There is no evidence to suggest that any specific routine screening intervention is beneficial in this age group but normal consultations with members of the practice team should provide the opportunity to encourage and arrange uptake of appropriate immunisations and for routine checks on visual acuity and hearing, and mental and physical development. Regular visits to dentist and optometrist should also be started. Screening for iron deficiency anaemia may be useful in at-risk groups including certain ethnic minorities and the socially deprived but we do not consider this should be done routinely.

Adolescence is often a difficult period of life when individuals tend to visit their family doctor infrequently but may nonetheless have unexpressed worries about their health and development. In the core programme of screening in general practice or at school, the only possible candidate for routine screening would be for immunity to rubella in girls. We would suggest that efforts would be more constructively aimed at improving awareness of the potential dangers of the virus in pregnancy and providing immunisation as necessary. However, every opportunity should be taken to provide appropriate information on lifestyle, risks to and care of health, and regular visits to the dentist and optometrist should be encouraged. Stress and psychiatric disorder are an important problem at this age but there is at present no satisfactory test available. Ways of tackling this do need attention as indicated in Chapter 4.

In adult men, the core programme of screening by the general practitioner should include screening for risk factors of coronary heart disease during normal surgery consultation. These factors should include weight, family history, cigarette smoking and blood pressure routinely, with measurement of cholesterol level if indicated. Again in normal consultation simple screening can be carried out for health damaging habits such as smoking, and drug or alcohol abuse. In the risk categories there should be appropriate worksite screening if necessary. One area that does require attention in this group, as in others, is screening for psychiatric disorders including depression but at present no satisfactory screening test exists. In adult women screening should take the same case-finding approach with the addition of the national screening programmes for cervical and breast cancer fully discussed in Chapter 6. We would reiterate here the possibility of considering joint breast/cervical cancer screening in the age group to which both apply.

The main aim of screening in old age is to identify disabilities that reduce the quality of life, as discussed in Chapter 7. Thus we would suggest that the programme of screening to be carried out mainly by general practitioners, health visitors, and social workers would include checks of general function such as sight, hearing, and mobility. There should be provision for attention from a chiropodist. There is also scope for attention to psychiatric depressive symptoms although as already stated there is no simple generally accepted screening test available. Other conditions for which screening in this age group should be considered if indicated are anaemia and hypertension, and problems such as social isolation should be addressed.

For such a national programme of screening to work effectively, there are various basic requirements and while these have already been covered earlier in the book, they bear repetition here.

In the first place, more adequate population registers must be devised. The registers being used for cervical cancer screening and breast cancer screening, for example, are the lists of names and addresses of general practitioners' patients, the shortcomings of which have been recently discussed (Bowling and Jacobson 1989; Armstrong 1989) and are fully dealt with in Chapter 6. The importance of an accurate data base is fundamental to the success of any screening programme and cannot be overemphasised.

Secondly, we need to know more about the availability of local diagnostic and treatment facilities than currently appears to be the case. This will require a systematic and thorough examination of each local area and is closely linked to another vital requirement—that of having one senior person in each health authority or board responsible for the co-ordination of all screening activities. This is one critical factor, more than almost any other, that emerges from a study of current screening literature. We have already stressed its importance very forcibly, particularly in discussion of the failure of the cervical cancer screening programme, and there are signs that health authorities are beginning to act—the Greater Glasgow Health Board, for example, has recently appointed a Director of Health Promotion. When, as is often the case, various different types of health professional are involved in a screening programme, co-ordination and communication can be at risk. The appointment of one senior person responsible for the programme and accountable for its successful organisation, implementation, and evaluation should minimise that risk.

Thirdly, there is a need to be much more rigorous about the establishment of national screening programmes to avoid the mistakes made, for example, at the start of the programme for cervical cancer screening. Proper evaluation must be built into any new proposal for screening and pressure from particular groups without supporting scientific evidence must be resisted.

There should, we suggest, be a small national advisory group, free as far as possible from political and professional pressure, to monitor and evaluate new proposals for screening and ongoing screening programmes. The Joint Sub-Committee on Screening in Medical Care was set up in 1968 as a sub-committee of the Standing Medical Advisory Committee (SMAC) to the Department of Health and Social Security and Welsh Office and of the Scottish Health Services Planning Council. This did look at new proposals for screening and reported to the Secretary of State for Health. However, it was disbanded by SMAC in 1981. The current position is that 'screening proposals are considered in the context of the particular area of medicine within which they fall and advice is sought from particular bodies and individual experts as appropriate'. This is too vague and indefinite a remit to be useful and leaves open the possibility of a particular screening proposal being espoused by either the enthusiasts or the sceptics. What we must aim for is reasoned consideration of any new proposal, taking account of recent scientific evidence across a broad base of professional opinion.

Fourthly, there should be a set of national priorities, objectives, and standards for health and health care. This is a complex and difficult area but one that must be tackled. The World Health Organisation objective of Health for All by the Year 2000 is well known and expressed in a number of specific targets. The American list of National Health Objectives reproduced as Table 2 in Chapter 1 seems perhaps too general and overstated but it exists and provides at least a crude yardstick by which to judge progress.

The Health Education Authority in England has

recently published its strategy for the next five years (HEA 1989). An independent multi-disciplinary committee has also designated 11 priority areas in public health which should help towards the attainment of what they see as three overall health goals—longevity, good quality of life, and equal opportunities for health (Smith and Jacobson 1988).

We would suggest a simple statement of four basic national health objectives for Britain in the 1990s.

1. To improve lifestyle and try to reduce health-damaging behaviour through effective health education and risk counselling to increase awareness of how individuals can improve and protect their own health.

2. To reduce environmental health hazards including those concerned with particular occupations.

3. To seek to control and reduce infectious diseases through an effective immunisation programme.

4. To apply presently effective and develop other simple screening tests which will identify individuals with a symptom or condition at a time when that symptom or condition is reversible.

To achieve these objectives we need more effective health promotion and health education. We must also always be aware of the possible dangers of screening as well as the concepts of benefit or no effect and beware of giving the impression that screening *per se* is beneficial. As the introduction to the US Preventive Services Task Force Report states

> physicians and other medical providers are well advised to be more selective in ordering screening tests, since their inappropriate use is at best wasteful and at worst harmful.

Fifthly, we must face the crucial question of finite resources. With increasing technological progress in diagnostic and other techniques at all stages of life, and perhaps particularly in the antenatal and neonatal periods, what should be available on the National Health Service and what should be personally financed? Are we reaching the stage where we do have to face the division of health care into ordinary and luxury?

This is an emotive area and one which health professionals are often reluctant to discuss. However it cannot continue to be shirked. Ellman (1989) raised the issue recently in a discussion of screening for breast cancer. As already mentioned in Chapter 6, she believes that frankness is vital and if it is stated clearly that screening without charge is being offered to provide a reasonable but not the maximum degree of protection against later development of advanced cancer and that extra screening at a financial cost can be offered to those who wish it, 'we may be able to promote more realistic expectations'.

Another possible approach would be to provide free of charge screening tests of proven efficacy while introducing a fee for tests which people choose to undergo but for which evidence of effectiveness is lacking. This can be illustrated by the example of screening for two of the main risk factors for coronary heart disease—blood pressure and cholesterol level. Raised blood pressure is a factor for which there is a simple reliable diagnostic test and provenly effective treatment. Cholesterol is also undoubtedly associated with the development of coronary heart disease. However, the contribution that a reduction in cholesterol level would make to CHD prevention is ambiguous and likely to be far less than that achieved by lowering blood pressure, stopping smoking, or reducing excess weight. A national food policy to reduce fat intake—for example, by encouraging people to eat less butter, skimmed rather than whole milk, and lean meat—would also undoubtedly have a beneficial effect in reducing mortality from CHD. Testing for raised blood cholesterol in Britain is also of dubious benefit when at least half the population are thought to have levels considered abnormal. Drug treatment has not yet been going on for long enough for its long-term efficacy to be established. It could, therefore, be argued that a test for blood pressure should be provided routinely and without charge as should dietary advice, while cholesterol testing and subsequent drug treatment should be subject to a fee until or unless scientific evidence of its efficacy becomes available.

Finally, we must emphasise the strong links between behaviour and health. In the late twentieth century any improvement in mortality is likely to come from improved control of behavioural risk factors such as cigarette smoking, alcohol consumption, poor or faulty nutrition, and lack of exercise. There is also a conflict between the individual and the state which it will be very difficult to resolve. Should we be attempting to introduce national guidelines in matters such as cigarette smoking or sugar consumption, or should we leave it to individuals to make their own decisions about their personal lifestyle and behaviour and its effects on their health. Obviously when lifestyle habits may damage the health of others as, for example, historically with tuberculosis and currently with HIV and cigarette smoking, the policy implications are clear.

We must have an honest debate about the future of screening and how it can be used constructively as a tool to improve the health of the population with a more unified and standard approach over the whole country, rather than being left to develop haphazardly and dependent on political and pressure group whim.

What is required overall is a comprehensive system of prevention, treatment, and care which must be adequately co-ordinated and available to all. This is of general relevance in our health service which is becoming more fragmented. Screening in the modern context should no longer be a discrete activity undertaken by a variety of individuals and authorities but instead should be part of a unified, national strategy for health. Screening is merely one aspect of health care provision—it must be linked to primary prevention including immunisation, it must be linked to appropriate health education, and it must be linked to adequate easy access to effective treatment. The most satisfactory method of screening in most cases will be to make use of the normal doctor-patient consultation to carry out the screening programme appropriate to the age and sex of the particular patient. However the complexities of this approach must not be underestimated, resource implications must be fully taken into account, and the support and participation of other practice staff will be vital.

In order to achieve maximum benefit cost-effectively, screening today has certain basic requirements which have been discussed throughout this book and which can be briefly summarised.

Firstly, there must be one senior person in each local health authority to co-ordinate screening activities.

Secondly, there must be satisfactory population registers with call/recall facilities in every general practice.

Thirdly, the screening process must be adapted to the needs of the specific population within nationally agreed guidelines. As Massie (1988) among others has pointed out the problem of providing health care is not the same in the highlands of Scotland as in the centre of London and there is a danger in over-simplifying the complexity of the National Health Service.

Fourthly, the previous criteria for screening, detailed in Chapter 1, must be observed, including the fact that there must be effective treatment available.

Fifthly, there must be proper evaluation of existing screening procedures and screening must be subject to medical audit.

Finally, a body should be established with overall responsibility for screening policy and specific responsibility for identifying screening procedures to be included in routine health care programmes and those which should be available only on request and possibly on payment of a charge.

Our overall aim for the next decade must be to ensure that screening is used effectively with good organisation and scientific evaluation so that it proves to be a benefit rather than a bane to the health of the population.

REFERENCES

ARMSTRONG, E. M. 'The politics of inadequate registers'. *Br Med J* 1989, 299:73.

BOWLING, ANN AND JACOBSON, BOBBIE. Screening: the inadequacy of population registers. *Br Med J* 1989, 298:545–6.

D'SOUZA, MICHAEL. 'Can I prevent disease and disability?' In *Epidemiology in General Practice.* D. MORRELL (ed.) Oxford: Oxford Medical Press, 1988.

ELLMAN, RUTH. Letter: 'Breast Cancer; a Response to Dr Maureen Roberts'. *Br Med J* 1989, 299:1337–8.

HALL, DAVID M. B. (ed.) *Health for All Children: a Programme of Child Health Surveillance.* Report of the Joint Working Party on Child Health Surveillance. Oxford: Oxford University Press, 1989.

HEALTH DEPARTMENTS OF GREAT BRITAIN. *General Practice in the National Health Service. The 1990 Contract.* London: Health Departments of Great Britain, 1989.

HEALTH EDUCATION AUTHORITY. *Strategic Plan 1990–1995.* London: Health Education Authority, 1989.

HELZLSOUER, K. Personal communication, 1990.

MASSIE, ALLAN. *How Should Health Services be Financed? A Patient's View.* Aberdeen: Aberdeen University Press, 1988.

SHAPER, A. G. Personal communication 1989—comment on the National Audit Office Report entitled *National Health Service: Coronary Heart Disease.*

SMITH, ALWYN AND JACOBSON, BOBBIE. *The Nation's Health. A Strategy for the 1990s.* London: King Edward's Hospital Fund for London, 1988.

US PREVENTIVE SERVICES TASK FORCE. *Guide to Clinical Preventive Services.* Baltimore: Williams and Wilkins, 1989.